Radiology of the Spine

Tumors

Edited by L. Jeanmart

With Contributions by

D. Baleriaux · M. Bard · P. Capesius · L. Divano
J. Frühling · D. C. Harwood-Nash · L. Jeanmart
M. C. Kaiser · J. D. Laredo · M. Lemort · J. J. Merland
D. Reizine · M. C. Riche · G. Sandt · M. Stienon

With 185 Figures

Springer-Verlag
Berlin Heidelberg New York Tokyo

Professor Dr. Louis Jeanmart

Service de Radiodiagnostic
Institut Jules Bordet
Centre des Tumeurs de l'Université Libre
de Bruxelles
Rue Heger-Bordet 1

1000 Bruxelles, Belgium

ISBN 978-3-642-49305-8 ISBN 978-3-642-49303-4 (eBook)
DOI 10.1007/978-3-642-49303-4

Library of Congress Cataloging-in-Publication Data. Main entry under title: Tumors (Radiology of spine) Includes bibliographies and index. 1. Spine — Tumors — Diagnosis. 2. Spine — Radiography. 3. Spinal cord — Tumors – Diagnosis. 4. Spinal cord — Radiography. I. Jeanmart, L., 1929- . II. Baleriaux, D. III. Series. [DNLM: 1. Spinal Cord Neoplasms. 2. Spinal Neoplasms. 3. Spine — radiography.
WE 725 T9245] RC280.S72T86 1985 616.99'2 85-17324
ISBN 978-3-642-49305-8

Softcover reprint of the hardcover 1st edition 1986

Reproduction of the figures: Gustav Dreher GmbH, Stuttgart

2127/3130-543210

Contents

Spinal Cord Tumors
D. Baleriaux. With 17 Figures

Spinal Neurinomas
G. Sandt, M.C. Kaiser, and P. Capesius. With 5 Figures

Spinal Tumors in the Child
D.C. Harwood-Nash. With 12 Figures

List of Contributors

D. Baleriaux, Department of Neuroradiology, Erasmus Hospital, Université Libre de Bruxelles, 1000 Bruxelles, Belgium

M. Bard, Hôpital Lariboisière, 2, rue Ambroise-Paré, 75010 Paris, France

P. Capesius, Department of Neuroradiology, Centre Hospitalier de Luxembourg, 4, rue Barblé, 1225 Luxembourg, Luxembourg

L. Divano, Institut Jules Bordet, Centre des Tumeurs de l'Université Libre de Bruxelles, Rue Heger-Bordet 1, 1000 Bruxelles, Belgium

J. Frühling, Institut Jules Bordet, Laboratoire des Radio-Isotopes, Service de Radiothérapie, Université Libre de Bruxelles, 1000 Bruxelles, Belgium

D.C. Harwood-Nash, Department of Radiology, Hospital for Sick Children, Toronto M5G 1X8, Canada

L. Jeanmart, Institut Jules Bordet, Centre des Tumeurs de l'Université Libre de Bruxelles, Rue Heger-Bordet 1, 1000 Bruxelles, Belgium

M.C. Kaiser, Department of Neuroradiology, Centre Hospitalier de Luxembourg, 4, rue Barblé, 1225 Luxembourg, Luxembourg

J.D. Laredo, Hôpital Lariboisière, 2, rue Ambroise-Paré, 75010 Paris, France

M. Lemort, Institut Jules Bordet, Centre des Tumeurs de l'Université Libre de Bruxelles, Rue Heger-Bordet 1, 1000 Bruxelles, Belgium

J.J. Merland, Hôpital Lariboisière, 2, rue Ambroise-Paré, 75010 Paris, France

D. Reizine, Hôpital Lariboisière, 2, rue Ambroise-Paré, 75010 Paris, France

M.C. Riche, Hôpital Lariboisière, 2, rue Ambroise-Paré, 75010 Paris, France

G. Sandt, Department of Neurosurgery, Centre Hospitalier de Luxembourg, 4, rue Barblé, 1225 Luxembourg, Luxembourg

M. Stienon, Radiodiagnostic Service, Institut Jules Bordet, Centre des Tumeurs de l'Université Libre de Bruxelles, Rue Heger-Bordet 1, 1000 Bruxelles, Belgium

Technical Considerations in the Diagnostic Workup of Spinal Tumors

M. C. KAISER and P. CAPESIUS

Tumors of the spine can be detected through various radiologic appearances considered with reference to the clinical symptoms presented. Bone tumors are probably found primarily on plain radiographs of the spine even when the patient does not present any neurologic deficit. Radionuclide bone scanning is the primary screening method for vertebral involvement by metastatic disease and the main method for showing its distribution throughout the spine. Examination of the spine exclusively with CT in every case would be extremely expensive and time consuming. While plain films of the spine show vertebral destruction or sclerosis in patients with abnormal activity seen on radionuclide bone scans, CT allows precise anatomic localization as well as gross characterization of the abnormality. CT has proved to be of great value in precise determination of the extent of involvement of both the vertebral bodies and their posterior elements an in indicating the presence of encroachment upon the spinal canal or intervertebral foramina. Although a specific histological diagnosis cannot usually be made by CT alone, the lesion can be characterized as to whether it is cystic or solid, vascular or nonvascular, diffuse or sharply delimited. CT-guided biopsies can be performed.

Intraspinal (intramedullary, extramedullary, intradural-epidural) tumors are quite often not detected until the stage of acute medullary compression. Metrizamide myelography is very helpful in determination of the precise site and extent of the lesion. Secondary computerized metrizamide myelography (CTMM) is extremely important, to define the lesion's topography relative to neighboring nervous tissue structures and to complement the geographical coordinates. The CT scan should be performed 3–4 h after myelography to obtain homogenous dilution of the water-soluble contrast medium. Anatomic details may be blurred if the contrast agent is still too concentrated and hyperdense. For the same reason we stress the importance of plain CT scanning in cases where severe bone involvement is suspected. The contrast material often has the same CT density as bone, and the interface between tumor and bone may no longer be outlined on secondary CTMM.

Paravertebral soft tissue masses in the abdomen and thorax are currently best evaluated with CT in preference to any other diagnostic method, invasive or noninvasive. CT permits accurate cross-sectional analysis of the spine, its contents, and the surrounding soft tissues. This remarkable technique has minimized the need for complex motion tomography and has extended the diagnostic accuracy beyond that possible with conventional radiographic modalities.

Furthermore, electronic reconstructions in coronal, sagittal, or oblique planes can be generated from serial axial slices to give a three-dimensional display of the lesions (Figs. 1 and 2). In selected cases direct coronal images can be obtained either by sitting the patients inside the gantry aperture or, in the case of children under a general anaesthetic, by laying them in a lateral decubitus position (Fig. 3) [2, 9]. The direct coronal mode is advocated because in this mode scans are generated along the long axis of the body and contain more useful information per generated image than in the conventional axial mode (Fig. 4). Detail is sharper on direct coronal images than on reconstructions, and without further radiation dose penalty, which might be necessary for reconstructions based on serial axial slices. Anatomic details demonstrated along this plane are very similar to those encountered by the surgeon during the operative approach. Nuclear magnetic resonance can provide a multiplanar display of spinal lesions with no need

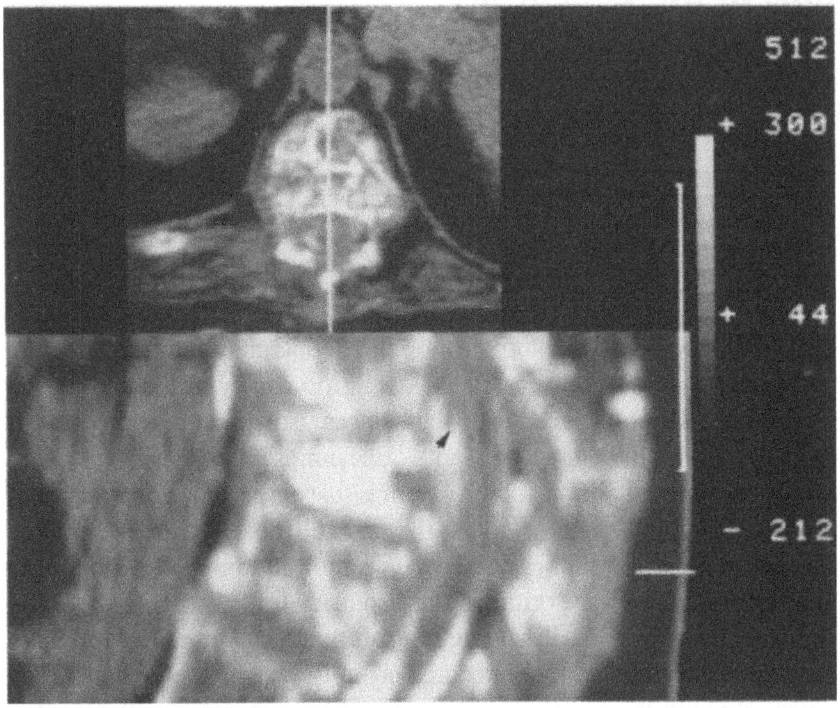

Fig. 1. Sagittal reconstruction in the upper lumbar region shows metastatic destruction of several vertebral bodies and kyphosis resulting from anterior vertebral compression. Intrathecal contrast medium is clearly outlined at the lower end of the reconstructed image. Intracanalar bone protrusion with compression of the cord can be recognized *(arrow)*. No intracanalar contrast medium is shown in the upper part of the vertebral canal, probably due to epidural tumor seeds. Note abdominal aorta anteriorly

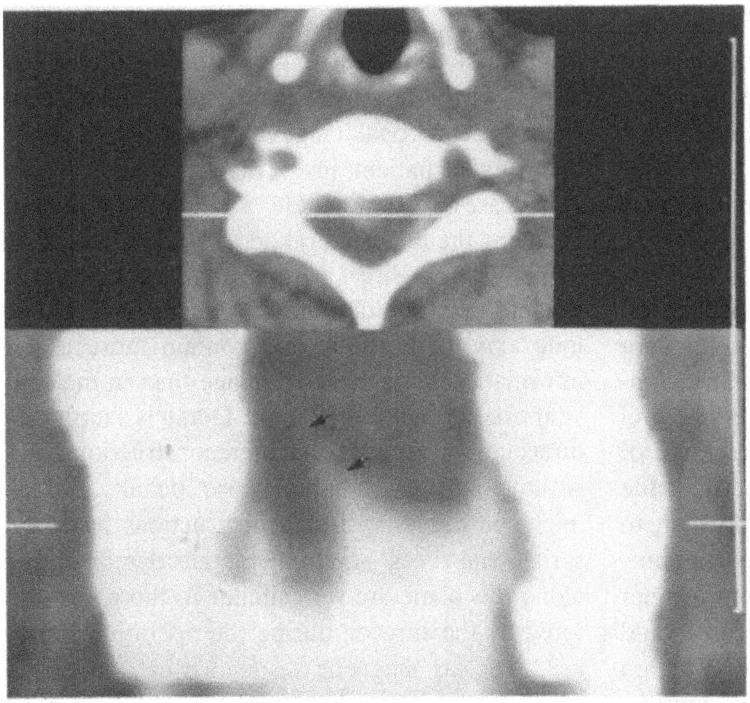

Fig. 2. Coronal reconstruction in the cervical region, showing large mass within the vertebral canal and displaced and compressed spinal cord *(arrows)*

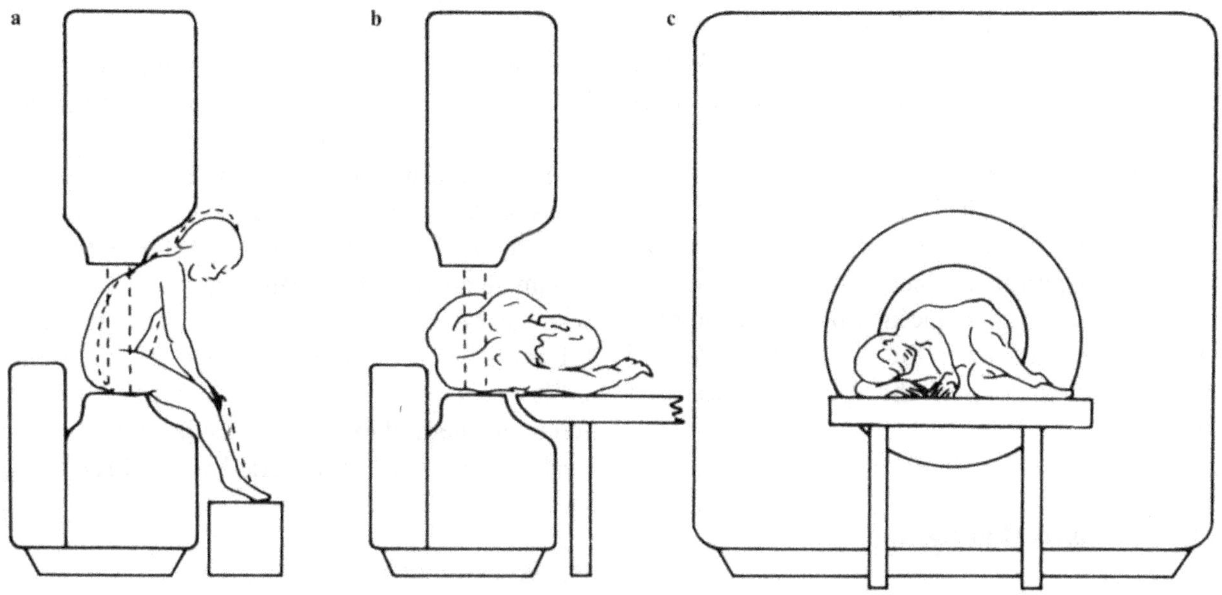

Fig. 3 a–c. Sitting position (**a**) and lateral position (**b, c**) for the direct coronal CT mode

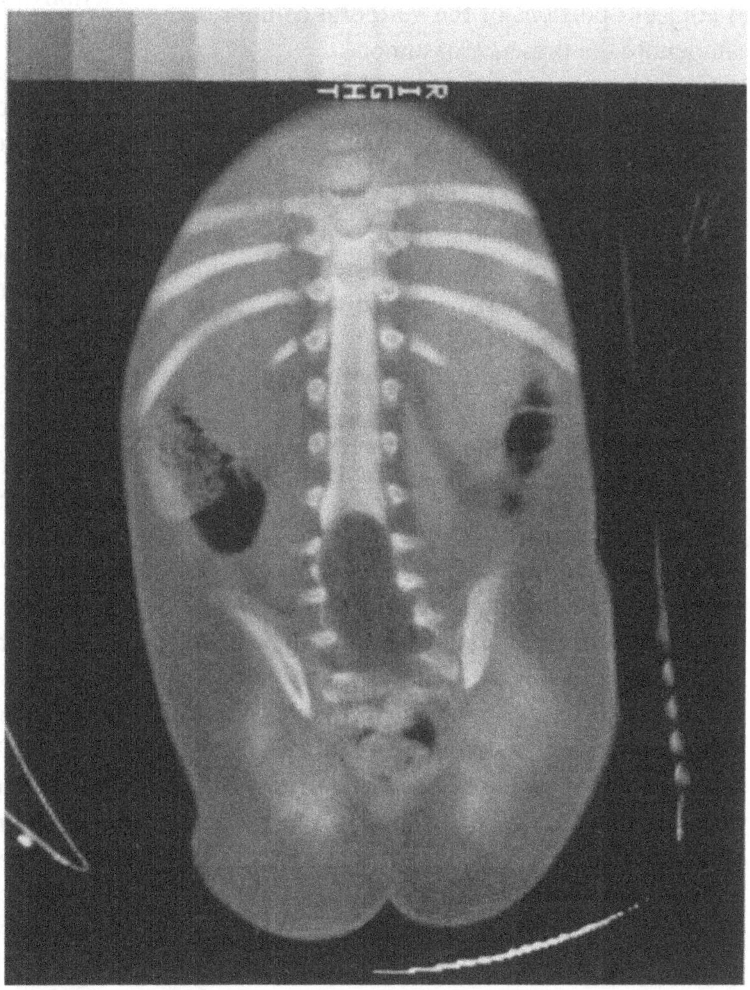

Fig. 4. Direct coronal image recorded in the lateral decubitus position in an infant under a general anesthetic. A long segment of cord and emerging nerve roots are outlined. At the level of the block, distal cord nerve roots are displaced by and intimately involved with a lipomatous mass [4]

to move the patient. Although it appears to be very promising for the diagnostic workup of intracanalar soft tissue abnormalities, this investigative mode has a rather limited capability for demonstrating bone pathology. In our opinion CT still remains the investigative procedure of choice for the evaluation of spinal tumors, as it shows bone and soft tissues equally well and only one visit to a radiology department is necessary.

The different radiologic investigation techniques and their application in the diagnostic workup of tumorous pathology of the spine are discussed below.

A. Standard Radiographs

As an outpatient procedure standard x-rays are very useful, as they provide a good indication of the location of spinal tumors. In plain roentgenograms of the spine there are several fundamental changes in adjacent portions of the vertebral column that can denote the presence of tumor:

1. Enlargement of the vertebral canal as manifested by flattening or concavity of the medial margins of the pedicle with an increased interpediculate distance, scalloping of the posterior vertebral wall, thinning of the lamina.
2. Enlargement of the intervertebral foramen resulting from tumor lying part within and part outside the spinal canal.
3. Calcifications within the tumor in the vertebral canal.
4. Osteolytic and/or osteosclerotic bone changes.
5. Paraspinal soft tissue thickening.

Although standard x-rays may provide important information about size, site, and extent of tumor pathology of the spine, the radiographic signs are late to become apparent, generally when neurologic signs of medullary compression are obvious. Whenever CT is not available, complex motion tomography may be required to obtain further details of any destruction and/or deformity of the vertebra and the size and shape of the vertebral canal, and to detect small intracanalar calcifications contained within the tumor.

I. Radionuclide Bone Scan

Radionuclide bone scanning is the primary screening method for detection of vertebral involvement by metastatic malignancy, particularly in cases where diffuse metastatic disease is suspected. In areas of abnormal activity CT examination may be carried out to provide definitive evidence of osseous involvement. This means that the radionuclide scan can be used as a guide preparatory to direct CT investigation to the precise site of the lesion. CT is too expensive and time consuming for use as a screening method for the entire spine, while radionuclide scans are easily carried out and relatively inexpensive.

II. Myelography

Several specific technical, radiologic, and clinical aspects of myelographic studies in tumor pathology of the spine are discussed below. Since the introduction of water-soluble contrast media it has been possible to explore the entire length of the vertebral canal in a single radiographic session. As a consequence, air myelography has practically disappeared from the investigation schedule for intraspinal tumors. The contrast material can be injected by the lumbar or the cervical route, by either a laterocervical or a suboccipital approach. We currently perform a laterocervical puncture between C1 and C2, but patients with neurologic deficit due to a neoplasm frequently cannot be placed in the prone position for cervical myelography. In these cases we position the patient on a tilting chair and use the suboccipital approach. The tilt of the chair should be adjusted in such a way that intracranial backflow of contrast medium is prevented. Whenever a total block to progression of contrast medium is found, the upper and lower limits of the neoplasm can be demonstrated by injecting contrast medium above and below the tumor during the same myelographic session (Figs. 5 and 6). It is generally conceded that the total volume of contrast medium injected can be much higher than for examinations where no block is found. The two solutions do not come in contact with each other because of the total block. When a tumor is present in the upper cervical region there may be a sudden intracranial backflow of the

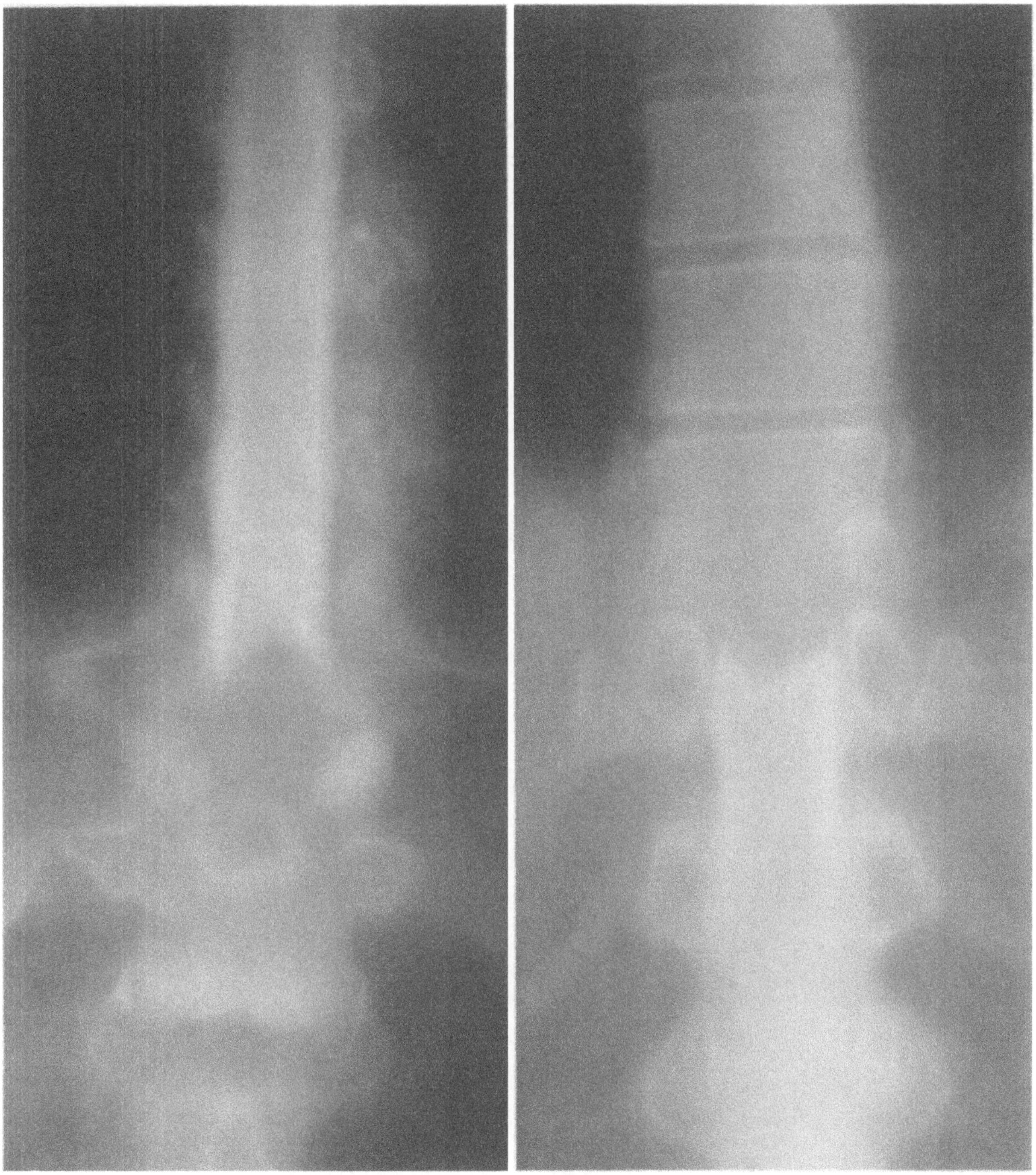

a b

Fig. 5 a, b. Total block due to intradural neurinoma, outlined by contrast injection from above and below the obstruction. A fairly precise demonstration of the shape, extension and topography of the tumor is obtained

contrast medium injected above the block. For this reason the injection of contrast medium should always be monitored by fluoroscopy. After the investigation the patient should stay in bed in an upright position for several hours.

If the lumbar puncture is performed beyond the level of a total myelographic block, typical spinal pain is provoked by the injection of contrast medium. This pain may be due to hypertension created by the actual injection. This pain in itself is

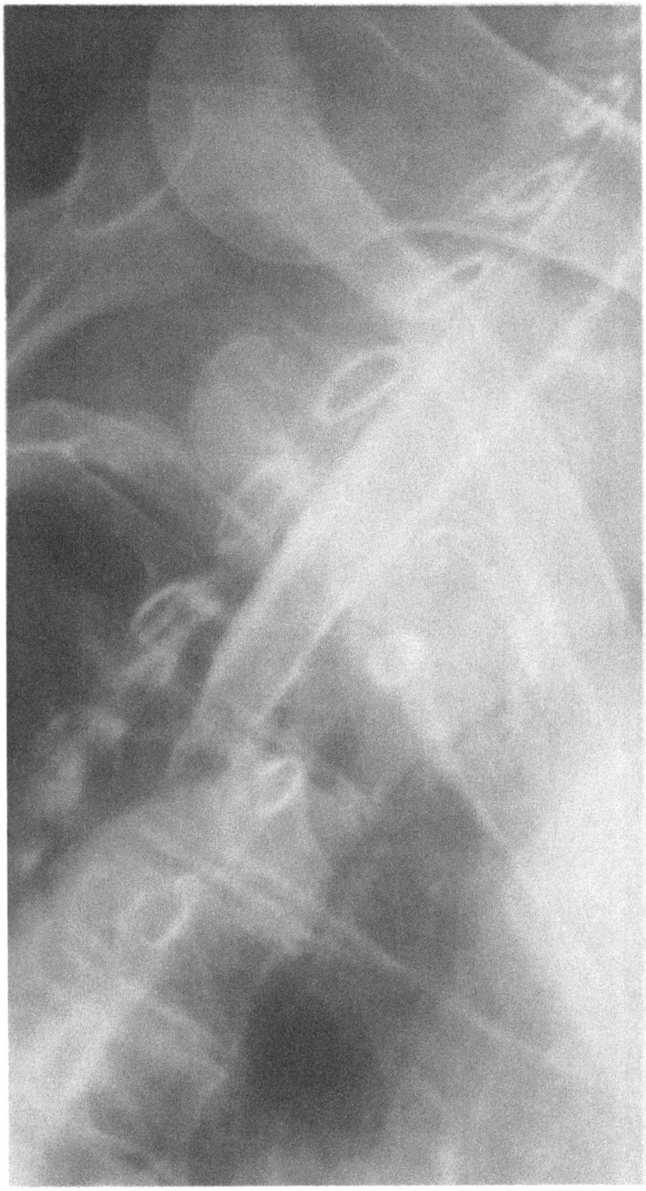

a

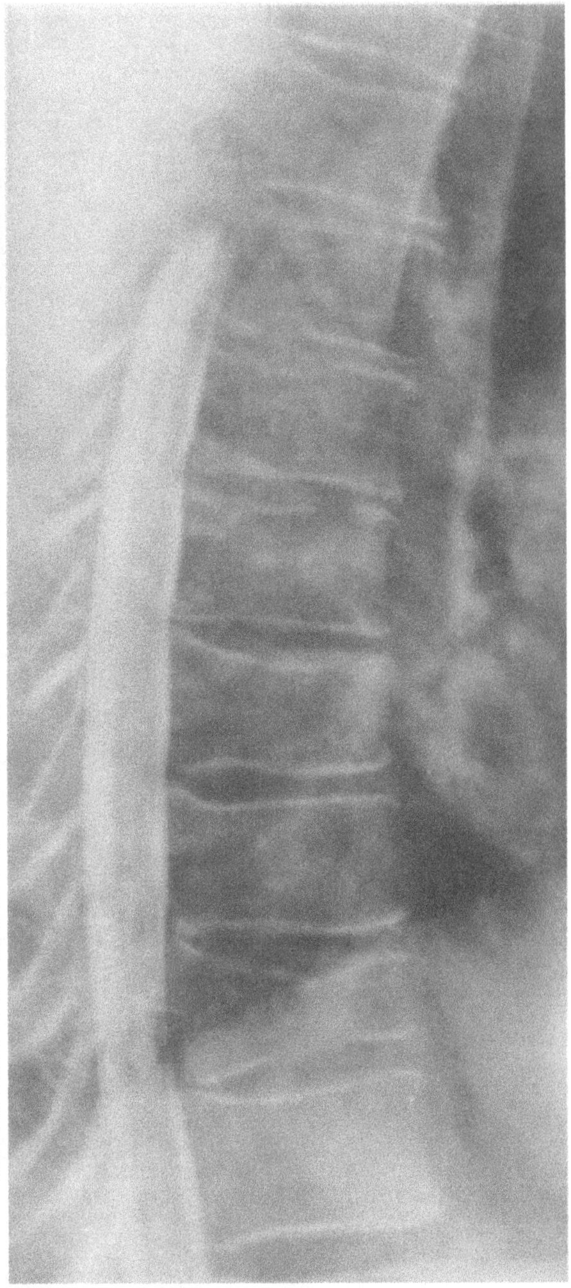

b

Fig. 6. a Oblique film of a cervical myelography shows obvious epidural thickening in the upper thoracic area owing to metastatic disease and a total block. This area can be shown with advantage on oblique films, as on lateral views the quality of images is impaired by overprojection of the shoulders. **b** Contrast injection by lumbar puncture shows the lower limit of the block caused by intraspinal metastatic disease

a strong indication that an intraspinal block is present.

In cases of subtotal or total block the clinical symptoms presented by the patient may worsen after the examination as hydrodynamic disturbances are created by the contrast medium. It is generally agreed that in cases where intraspinal tumor pathology is suspected myelography should only be performed in clinical centers where a neurosurgical team is on hand to perform any emergency interventions and where a close clinical followup after the investigation is assured.

There may be considerable technical and radiologic problems in attaining adequate visualization of the lower cervical and upper dorsal regions, owing to overprojection of the shoulder girdle. In many cases AP, and above all oblique, views are very much more informative than lateral pictures of the cervicodorsal junction (Fig. 6a). In many instances myelography provides a precise topographic localization of the tumor process: intramedullary/intradural and extramedullary/extradural. In some cases, however, the topographic diagnosis may be difficult, and secondary CTMM should be generated at the level of the tumor to complement the diagnostic and topographic information. The main advantage of CT over myelography is that it can demonstrate paravertebral (extraspinal) extension of the neoplasm if present.

III. Computed Tomography

To obtain optimal computed tomography (CT) images of the spine and intraspinal contents high-resolution scanners of the third and fourth generation are required; these need to have short scanning times and to accept a variety of software facilities allowing for multiplanar reconstructions. The information gained can be further enhanced through a special high-resolution or review program in which the raw data are processed to enhance the contrast and to increase spatial resolution. A lateral localizer image (scoutview or topogram) should be used to select the appropriate vertebral level and an adequate gantry angulation. The segment(s) of the spine to be examined by CT scan is are determined upon examination of standard x-ray films, radionuclide bone scan, and/or metrizamide myelography. CT scoutviews are generally underrated as diagnostic imaging modes, although they are almost routinely used for localization of vertebrae and disk spaces. It has been proved that bone lesions and some intracanalar soft tissue masses can be demonstrated with advantage by CT scoutviews [3]. A 2-mm slice thickness should be used in the cervical area, while a 4-mm slice thickness is sufficient in the thoracic or lumbar area. Whenever electronic reconstructions in the sagittal, coronal, and oblique planes are contemplated whole series of contiguous axial slices must be examined. All the CT images are electronically enlarged, and a double image display in conventional gray and reverse modes in combination with window manipulations is a further essential condition for high diagnostic accuracy. In selected cases direct coronal CT scanning can be achieved if the patient is seated within the gantry aperture and the height so adjusted that the region of interest is well enclosed within the circle of reconstruction. Pelvis and thighs must not be too close to the detectors, to prevent artefacts from high-density bony anatomic structures. This position can be achieved by sitting the patient either on the moving tabletop device or on a foam structure within the gantry aperture (Fig. 3). In the case of infants and small children under a general anesthetic the patient is placed in a lateral decubitus position with the head tucked in and the knees tucked up (Fig. 3) [2]. We used a 10-mm slice thickness and a 9.6-s scanning time. The largest circle of reconstruction must be used.

Reconstruction modes can be fairly accurate for diagnostic purposes, and they give a good idea of the geographic distribution of the lesions, but for management planning by means of radiotherapy or surgery the direct coronal mode offers more useful information overall than any other mode (Fig. 4).

For accurate diagnosis of intracanalar tumors intrathecal contrast medium must be injected, as tumor and nervous tissue have almost the same density and the various soft tissue components cannot be differentiated by plain CT. In most cases CT is performed as a secondary investigation following previous metrizamide myelography. Whenever significant bone involvement is suspected we recommend that plain CT should first be carried out, as the bone margins are best shown without intracanalar contrast medium. Some tumors may show enhancement after IV injection of contrast medium (neurinomas, meningiomas, hemangiomas) but the images are often not conclusive. Intramedullary tumors generally do not have an abnormal density and are isodense with the cord. For this reason diffuse cord swelling and small intramedullar tumors may not be recognized on plain CT scans. Myelography defines the level and extent of the process, while secondary CTMM shows up precisely what compressive mechanism and what structures are involved, and also reveals any tumor extension beyond and outside the verte-

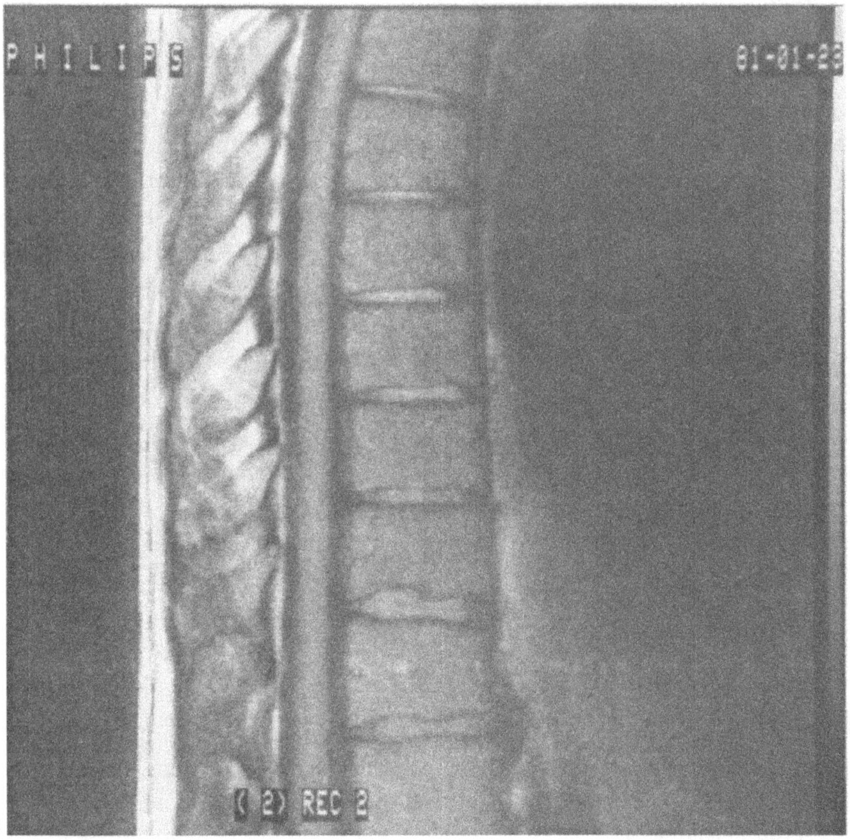

a

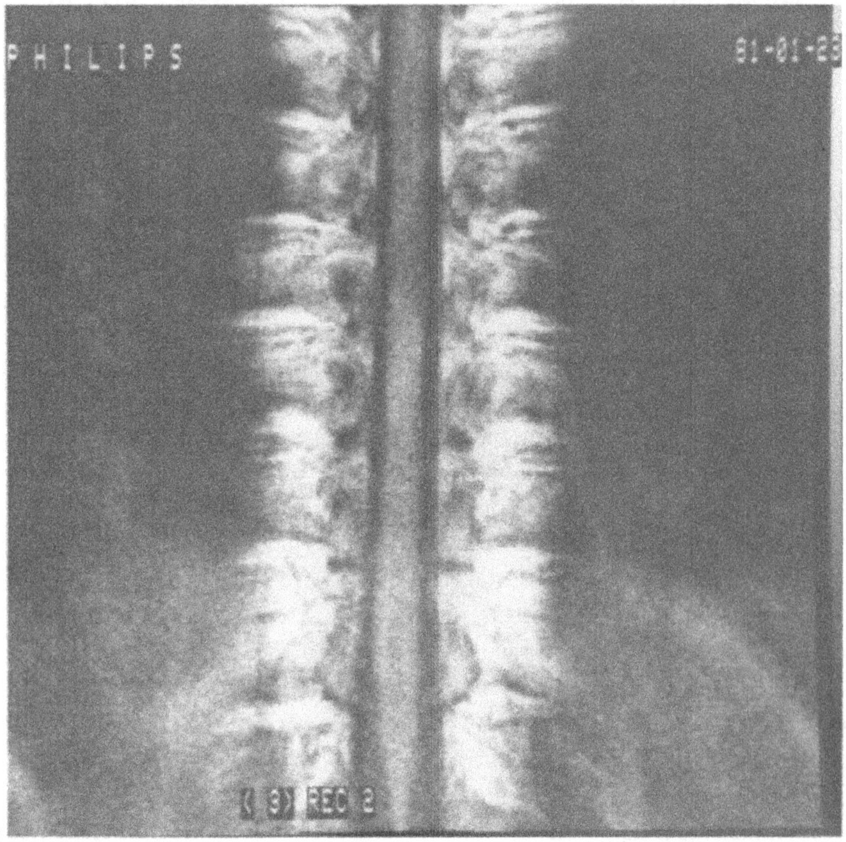

b

Fig. 7a, b. Magnetic resonance imaging: surface coil images recorded in an example of normal spinal cord. **a** Sagittal cut at midthoracic level; **b** normal coronal view of lower thoracic myelum and conus medullaris. These images were obtained with a 0.5 Tesla superconducting unit (Philips Gyroscan) bral canal. In some cases a delayed CT scan can reveal useful information such as opacification of a syringomyelic cavity secondary to a tumor.

IV. Special Procedures

In small children ultrasonography can be used for investigation of the lower lumbar canal. Sonographic windows are provided by the incomplete ossification of the immature posterior elements in children under 1 year of age and in spina bifida. Structural deformities of congenital anomalies can be displayed. It has been demonstrated that intraspinal masses (lipomas, teratomas, intramedullary dermoids) can be shown with advantage by high-resolution real-time sonography [6]. Real-time sonography reveals not only the nonradiopaque parts of the spinal column, such as cartilage, spinal cord, subarachnoid space, and nerve roots, but also vascular pulsations, and it permits rapid visualization of suspected pathology in the transverse and longitudinal planes.

Percutaneous needle biopsy of vertebral and paravertebral masses can be accomplished with both ease and accuracy if CT is applied for guidance in placement of the needle. Spinal cord angiography does not offer any advantage in the study of intramedullary tumors other than hemangioblastomas and adds nothing to the management of the patient [1]. Embolization of vascularized vertebral tumors can be carried out to facilitate surgery. But it can also be performed without subsequent operation in the case of vertebral hemangiomas and as a palliative measure in malignant neoplasms to reduce radicular or spinal cord compression syndromes [8].

The value of nuclear magnetic resonance (NMR) (Fig. 7) in the study of tumors within the vertebral canal and cord has still not been fully assessed, but it has the potential to be of a high value [5, 7]. Its sensitivity is very high, but the specificity still appears to be limited. With an appropriate pulse-sequence technique the spinal cord, brainstem, cerebrospinal fluid, and extradural structures such as the intervertebral disk can be outlined without the use of intrathecal contrast or ionizing radiation [5]. Its ability to image the cord directly, rather than indirectly as in myelography, the absence of bone artefacts such as are encountered with CT, and the multiplanar capabilities indicate that NMR will one day be the procedure of choice for evaluation of the cord and intracanalar contents [7].

References

1. Djindjian R, Hurth M, Houdart R (1971) Hémangioblastomes médullaires et maladie de von Hippel-Lindau. Travail préliminaire à propos de 14 cas étudiés par angiographie médullaire. Rev Neurol 124:495–502
2. Kaiser MC, Pettersson H, Harwood-Nash DC, Fitz CR, Armstrong E (1981) Direct coronal CT of the spine in infants and children. AJNR 2:465–466
3. Kaiser MC, Capesius P, Veiga-Pires JA, Sandt G (1984) A new sign of lumbar disk herniation recognizable on lateral CT scoutviews. Report on six illustrative and selected cases J Comput Assist Tomogr 8:1066–1071
4. Kangarloo H, Gold RH, Diament MJ, Boechat MI, Barrett C (1984) High-resolution spinal sonography in infants. AJNR 5:191–195
5. Modic MT, Weinstein MA, Pavlicek W, Boumphrey F, Starnes D, Duchesneau PM (1984) Magnetic resonance imaging of the cervical spine: technical and clinical observations. AJNR 5:15–22
6. Naidich TP, Fernbach SK, McLone DG, Shkolnik A (1984) Sonography of the caudal spine and back: congenital anomalies in children. AJNR 5:221–234
7. Norman D, Mills CM, Brant-Zawadzki M, Yeates A, Crooks LE, Kaufman L (1984) Magnetic resonance imaging of the spinal cord and canal: potentials and limitations. AJNR 5:9–14
8. Stoeter P, Voigt K (1980) Selective spinal angiography and embolization of tumors of the vertebral column. In: Veiga-Pires JA, Martins da Silva M, Oliva L (eds) Intervention radiology. Excerpta Medica, Amsterdam, pp 196–201
9. Veiga-Pires JA, Kaiser MC (1982) Direct coronal mode (DCM) in whole-body CT scanning. BJR 55:75–78

Primary Tumors of the Osseous Spine

M. Stienon and L. Jeanmart

A. Introduction

The differential diagnosis of tumorous lesions of osseous origin, particularly at the level of complex architectural structures such as the elements of the vertebral column, often poses difficult problems. The diagnosis must differentiate not only between the different primitive tumorous pathologies, but must also differentiate these from lesions of quite different natures, e.g., inflammatory and degenerative, and from overall metastatic lesions, which make up the vast majority of bony tumors of the spine and are often the first manifestation of primary neoplastic disease.

There are few absolute radiologic criteria that are pathognomonic for particular tumors, and the diagnosis of their nature is complicated even further by the polymorphism of the pathologic entities and the variability of clinical signs. In a substantial proportion of cases, the final diagnosis will rest with the pathologist, the clinical and the radiological data giving indications of the lesions' suspected nature. Computed tomography (CT), which has proved highly valuable in the diagnosis and the assessment of spread of tumors in the soft tissues and in the understanding of mechanical or compressive lesions of the vertebral column, is unfortunately not significantly more helpful than radiology in differential diagnosis. Its usefulness in the assessment of extension of the tumor remains important, and is even irreplaceable.

B. Genuine Tumors of Bony Origin

I. Osteoid Osteoma

Spinal osteoid osteomas, like those at other predilection sites, affect predominantly the male sex with a peak incidence in the 2 and 3 decades (age range 1–50 years).

Pain is virtually always present. Sometimes neurologic symptoms are the first indications of disease (e.g., a radicular pain pattern). The pain is classically worst at night and is relieved by aspirin.

The most frequent localization is the lumbar region, although all levels can be affected. The neural arch is preferentially affected: the spinous processes of the vertebrae, isthmuses, tranverse processes, and more rarely, the vertebral body (Figs. 1 and 2).

The lesions affecting the vertebral body originate in the cancellous bone, while those at the level of the posterior arch and the apophyses more often arise in the cortical bone.

The periosteal reaction is less pronounced than in the long bones, which makes identification difficult.

Scoliotic curvature with its peak deviation at the level of the lesion is often encountered. The nidus is hypervascular, transparent or sclerotic, and the peripheral scleral reaction is best visualized at the pedicular or apophyseal transverse process.

The lesions can be 3–4 cm in diameter, and spontaneous diminution in volume is sometimes encountered.

II. Osteoblastoma

This rare tumor (less than 1% of osseous tumors) preferentially affects the axis of the spine (about 40% of all cases).

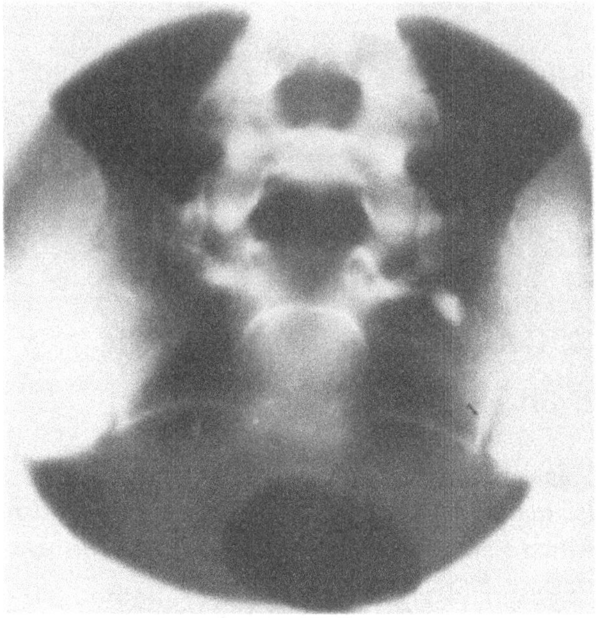

Fig. 1. Patient aged 29 years presented with nocturnal sacral pains. Osteocondensing lesion of the left pars lateralis was found to be an osteoid osteoma

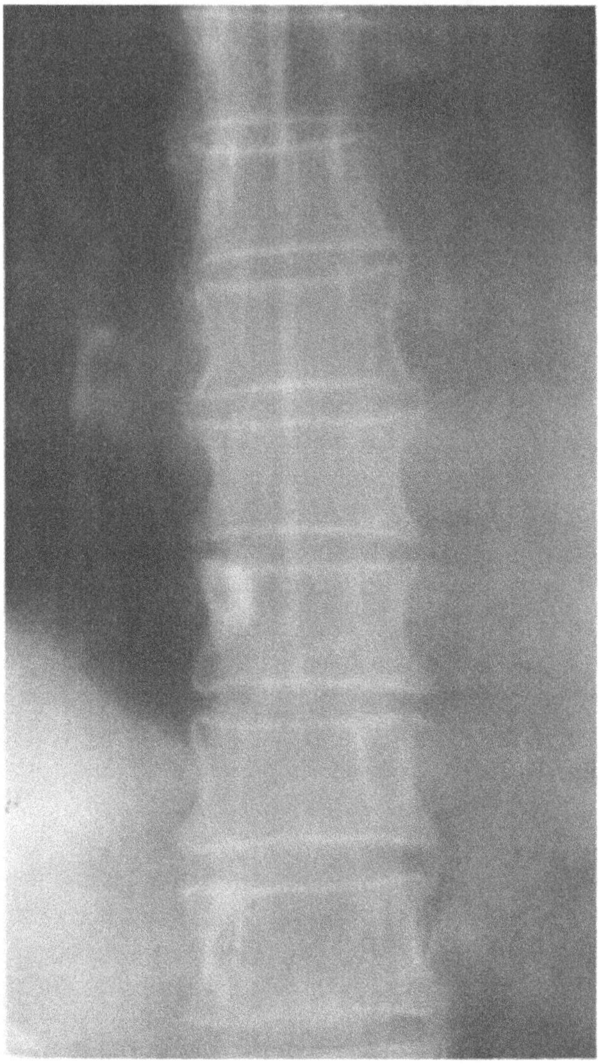

Fig. 2. Osteoid osteoma of the right pedicle of Th10

Its relationship, or even histologic identity, with osteoid osteoma is underlined by all authors; according to some, the size of the nidus seems to influence behavior of the adjacent tissue.

The incidence is maximum between the ages of 10 and 20 years (range 5–78 years), with a male predominance. The symptoms are pain, which is less characteristic than in the case of osteoid osteoma, worsens progressively, and is not amenable to aspirin. A mass can sometimes be palpated clinically. Radicular or myelocompressive syndromes, sometimes amounting to a complete block, can be encountered. Scoliosis, inverted curvature, and torticollis are frequent. The radiologic appearance is that of primary osteolytic tumors, which are radiotransparent with fine calcifications and can bring about destruction of the bone by breaking its cortical part. Amorphous calcifications are present but do not arise in the same manner as in the case of cartilaginous tumors. A fine calcic border, which is sometimes broken, surrounds the tumor in about half the cases (Figs. 3 and 4). There is no periosteal reaction. The vertebral body is rarely affected, the preferred sites being the neural arch and the spinous process (Figs. 5 and 6).

Reactive densification of the vertebral body is sometimes encountered.

The tumor is hypervascular (Fig. 6). Its appearance is sometimes aggressive, but metastases are

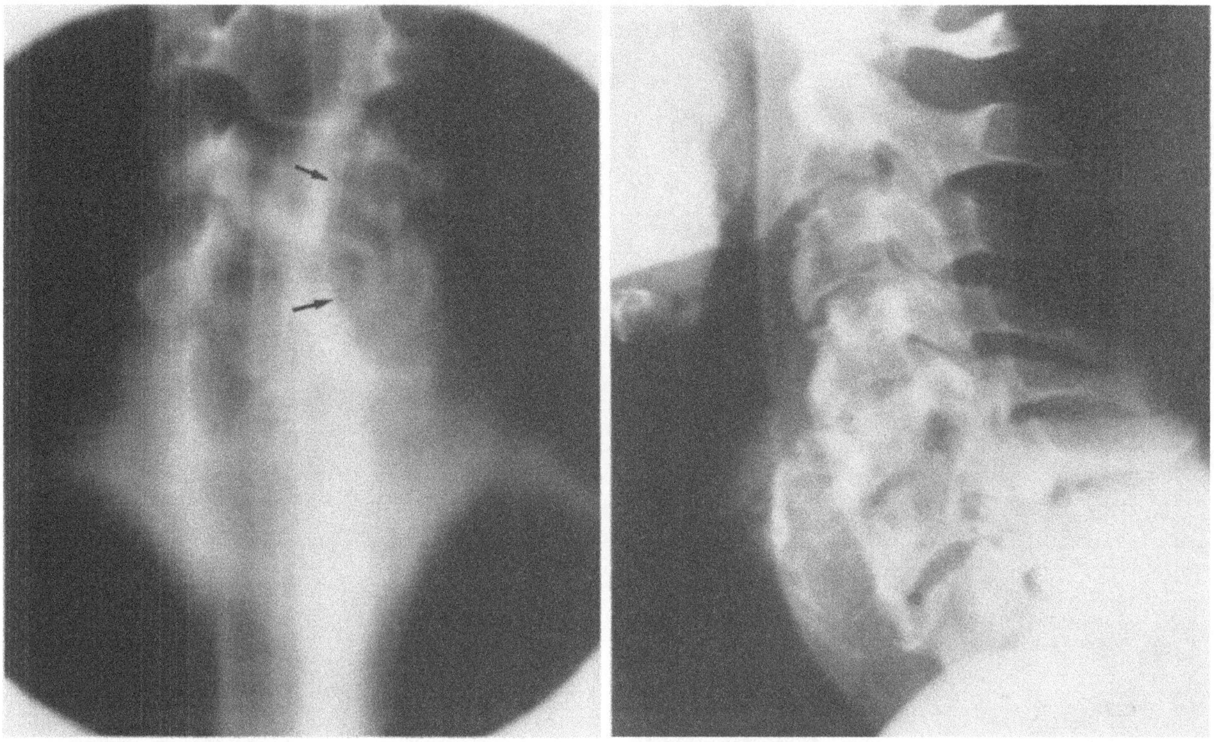

a b

Fig. 3 a, b. Tumor of C5–C6 discovered during a checkup for scoliosis in a man of 21 and biopsied. Lesion of the body of C5–C6 extending to the left at C6 towards the pedicle, the lateral mass, and the transverse process. Note the structure character of the tumor and the fine peripheral calcic border. **a** front-view tomogram; **b** standard roentgenogram

absent. However, transformation into osteosarcoma has been described. Recurrences also occur in about 10% of cases (Fig. 7). The treatment of choice is still surgery whenever it is possible, and when not, radiotherapy.

III. Bone Islands

These dense lesions are asymptomatic, appear at all ages, and can regress or grow spontaneously (not illustrated).

IV. Osteosarcoma

Osteogenic sarcomas are rarely (0.85%–2%) spinal: (1% in the series reported by Barwick et al.).

These lesions can be radiotranslucent (Figs. 8–10), strongly sclerosed or mixed with osseous neoformation extending toward the adjacent soft tissue.

Association with Paget's disease is frequent (Fig. 8) (3 cases out of 10 in the above-mentioned series; conversely, 3%–14% of patients with Paget's disease also have osteosarcoma. An association with anterior radiotherapy is also claimed. Differential diagnosis from osteoblastoma is difficult, although the age group and the more frequent origin at the level of the vertebral body than the posterior arch are good indicators. A particular form of the disease must be mentioned, viz, osteosarcomatosis, multiple condensing tumor, which affects children 5–10 years of age.

The preferred sites are the lumbar and sacral areas. In all cases the prognosis is uncertain. The treatment varies from one subject to another, total resection rarely being possible. Chemotherapy and radiotherapy are therefore preferred, and surgery is reserved for palliative or decompressive treatment.

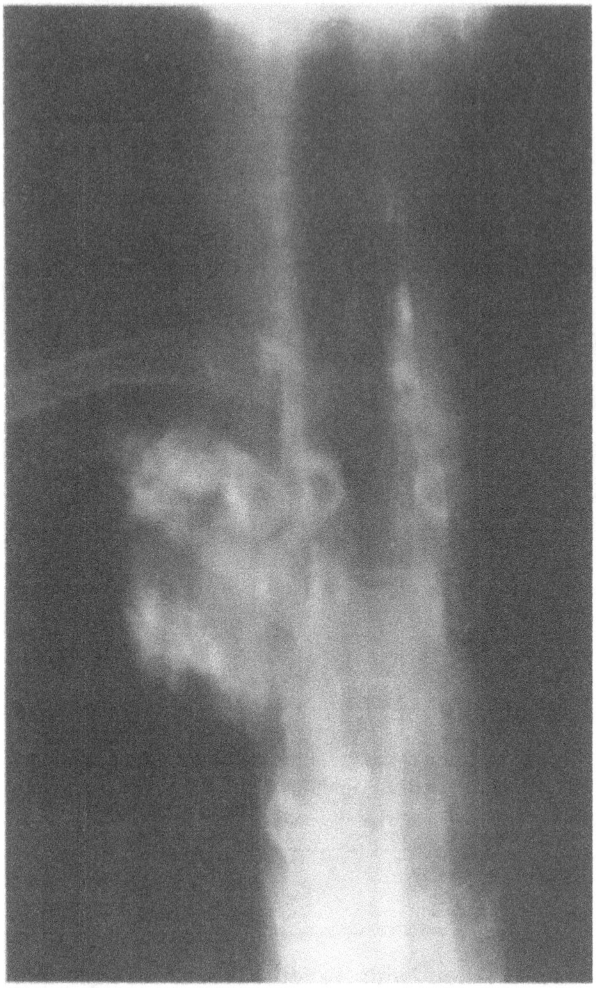

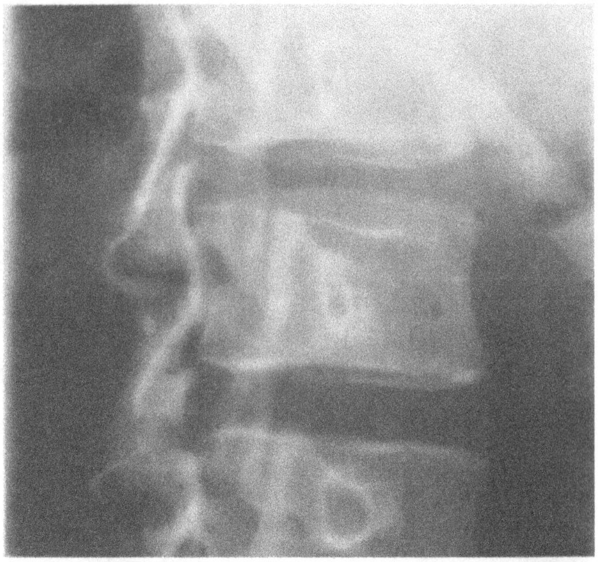

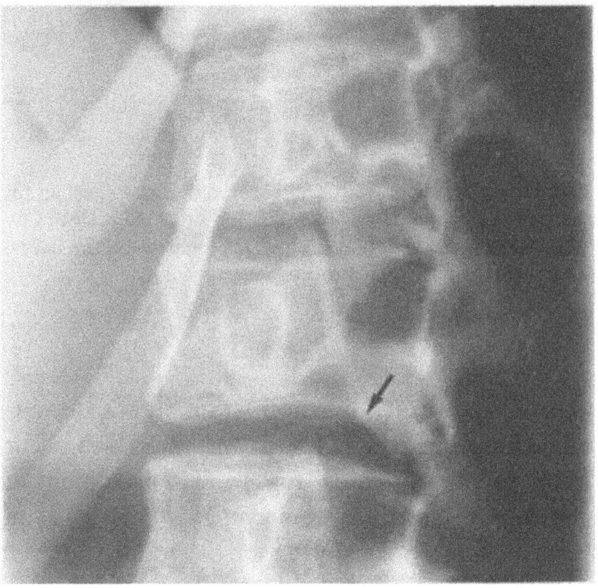

Fig. 4. Chondrosarcoma with laterovertebral extension at Th3, 4, and 5 in a 57-year-old woman. Note the irregular calcic density at the center of the tumor

Fig. 5. Osteoblastoma of the inferior para-articular process of Th12 with virtually complete lysis of the isthmus

V. Chondrosarcoma

Chondrosarcomas occur in the vertebral column. These lesions are slow-growing, extending in size over some years, and vascular. They originate in the vertebral body or in the posterior arch, and extension in to the perivertebral soft tissue or the vertebral canal is common. They can even affect many adjacent levels. Radiologically they are predominantly lytic, and they often contain irregular calcified dense spots.

VI. Osteochondroma

Benign cartilaginous tumors rarely occur in isolation, even apart from the syndrome of multiple hereditary exostosis. The predilection sites for implantation are anywhere in the posterior part of the vertebral column, the spinous process in particular but also the tranverse process (Fig. 11) and the vertebral lamina. Typically, continuity is observed between the cortical part of the healthy bone and that of the osteochondroma.

a 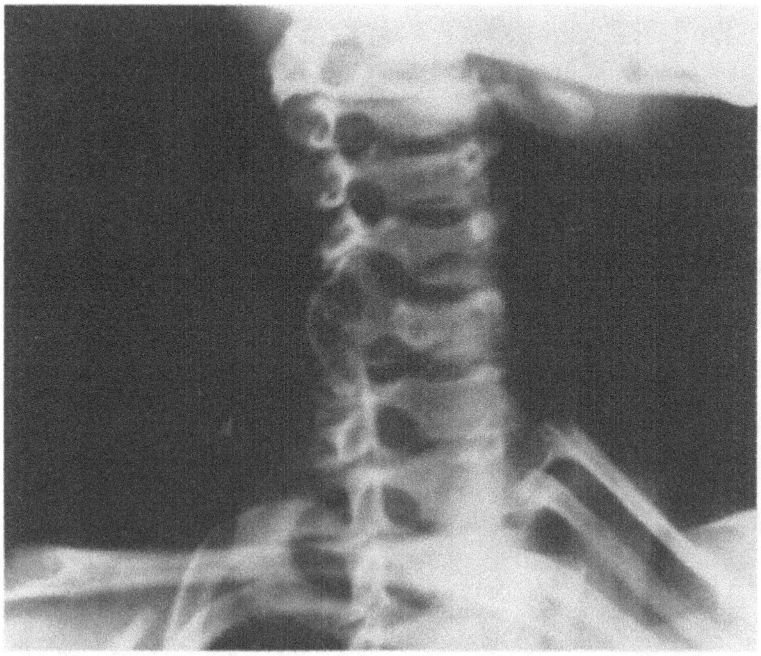 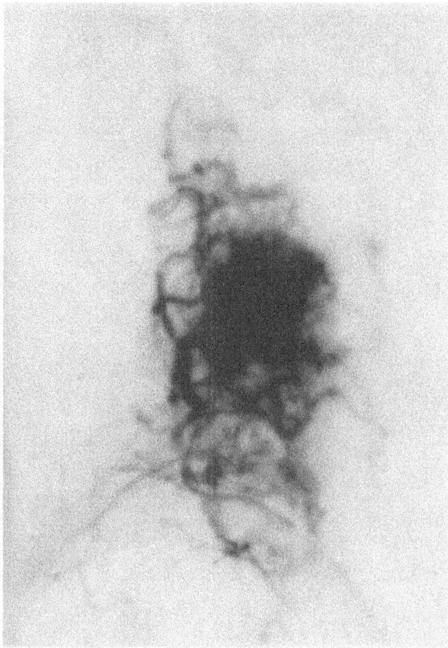 b

Fig. 6. a Girl 7 years old presented with cervical pains. Investigation revealed osteoblastoma involving the spinous process of C6 with articular deterioration. **b** Arteriography and embolization. Were performed

Transformation of this tumor into chondrosarcoma is possible (1 % of isolated forms, 10 %–15 % of familial forms).

VII. Osteoclastoma (Giant Cell Tumor)

The predilection site in the vertebral column is the sacrum, which is affected from two to seven times as often as the other segments affected by this tumor. The age group affected is approximately the same as that in which, peripher al tumors of this type arise, i.e., the 3 and 4 decades.

The lesion does not have a typical radiologic appearance. It is more often seen as a zone of thinning or of osseous destruction. The tumor is very highly vascularized and can extend to several adjacent levels.

Malignant transformation and degeneration into osteosarcoma are not rare (Figs. 12, 13).

VIII. Fibrosarcoma

Though rare in the spine, fibrosarcomas sometimes occur in sacral sites. They are seen as predominantly lytic lesions, with extension to the adjacent soft tissue.

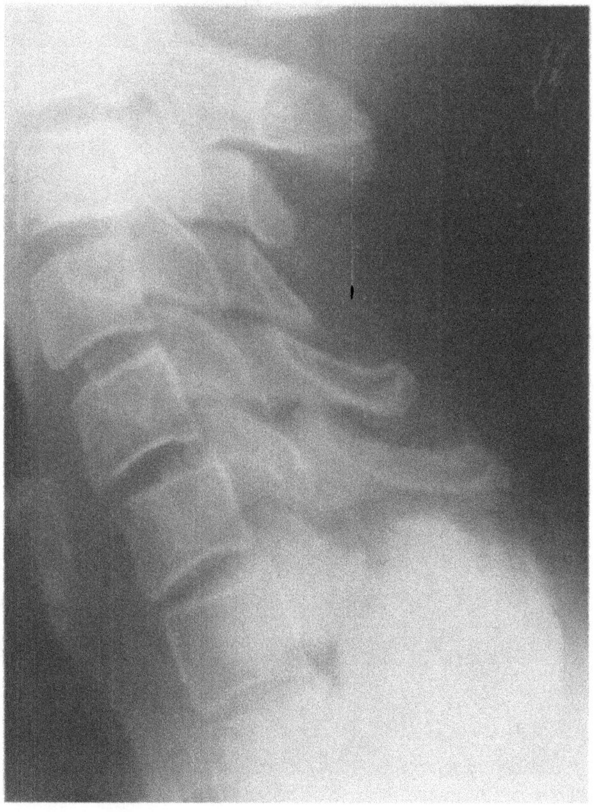

Fig. 7. Osteoblastoma of the spinous process of C7

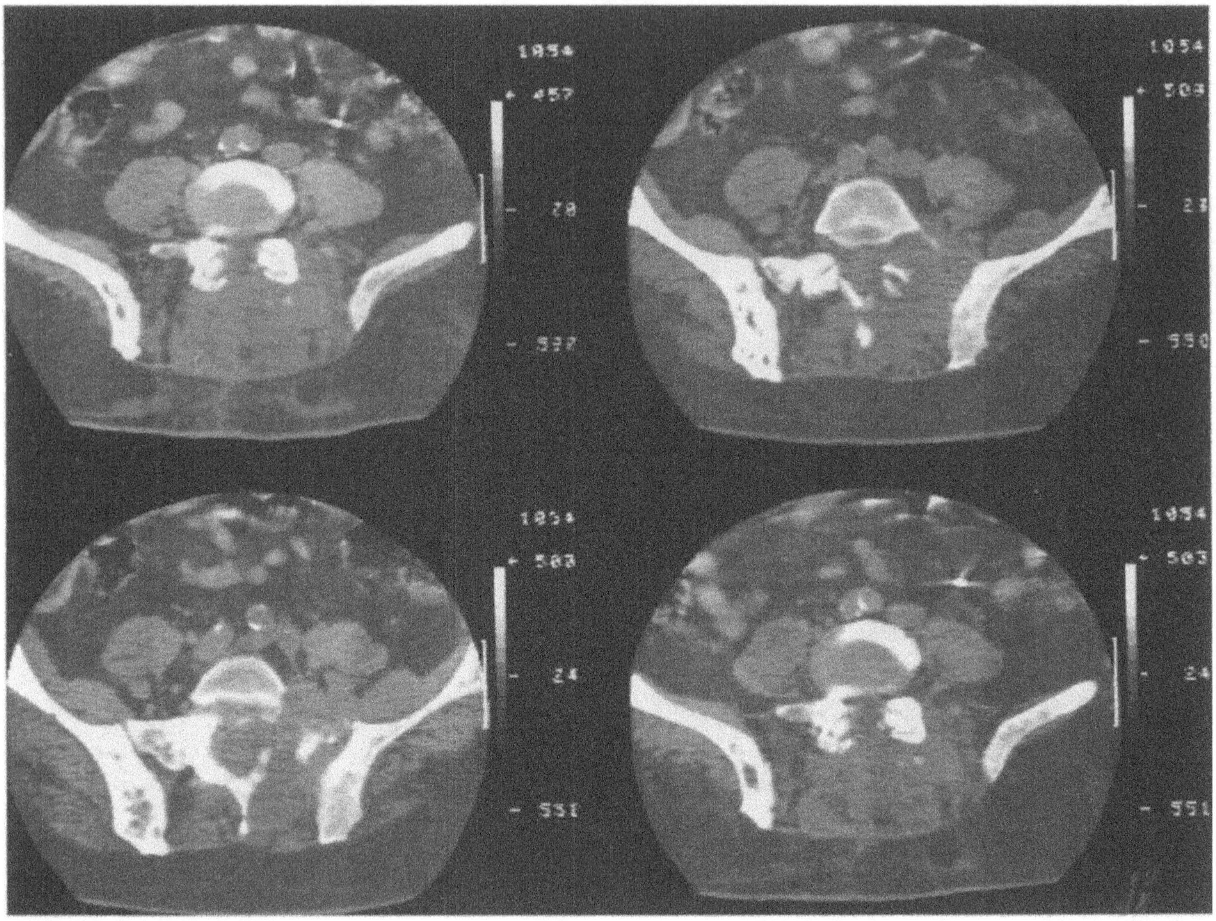

Fig. 8

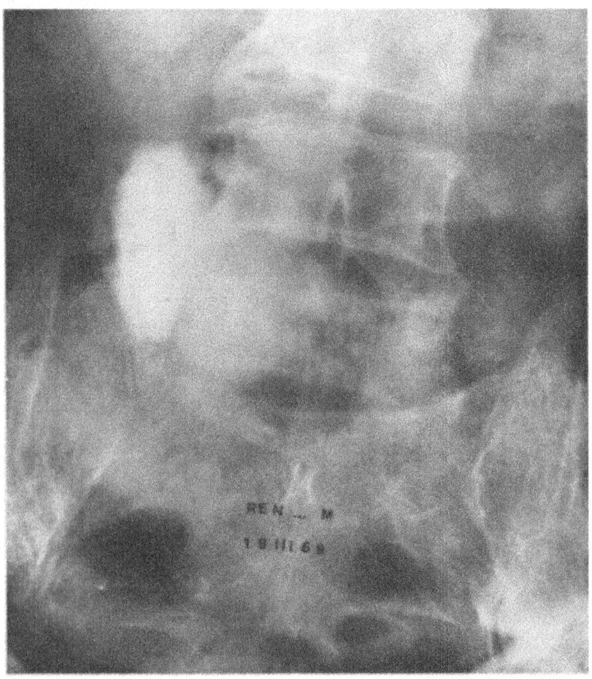

Fig. 9

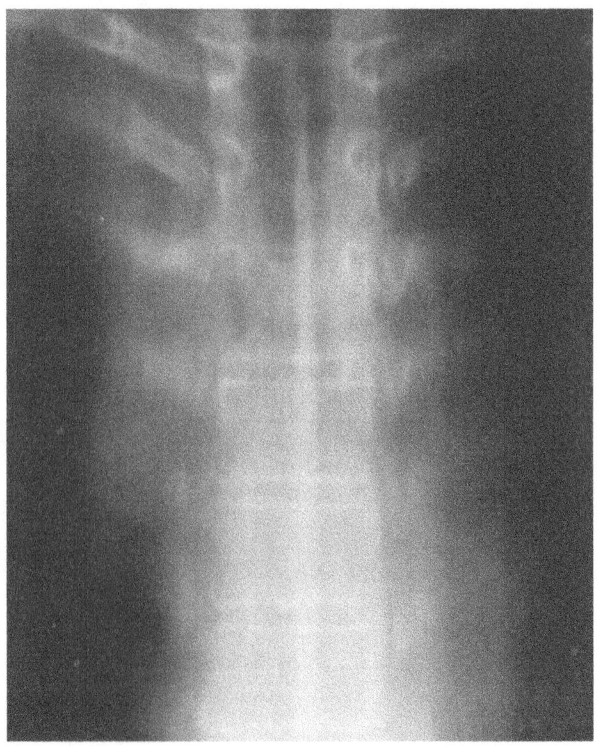

Fig. 10

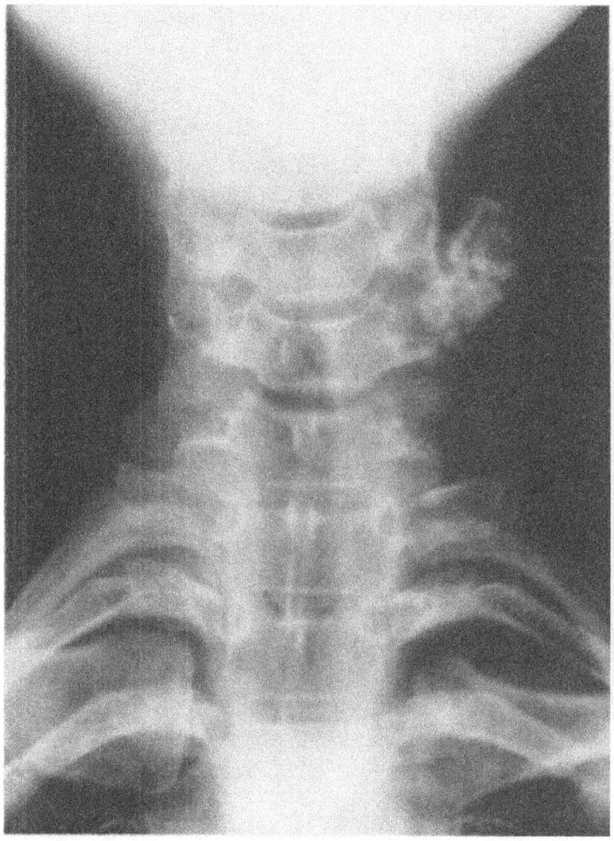

a

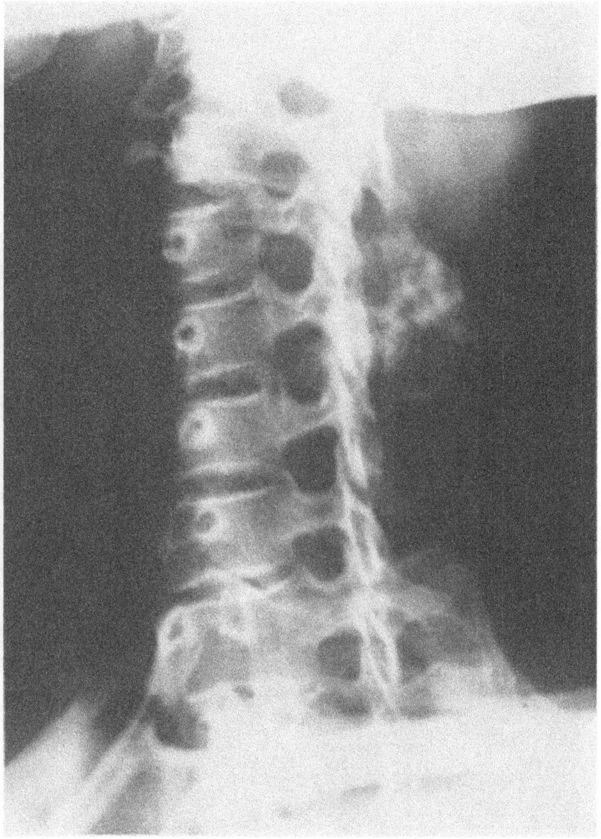

b

Fig. 11 a, b. Left cervical swelling in a 22-year-old woman. Exostosis of left fibula and tibia. Benign exostosis developed, of the transverse process at C5. Curative surgery. **a** Front view; **b** right anterior oblique view

◁ **Fig. 8.** CT with emboli revealing an osteosarcoma affecting L5 and S1, developed against a background of Paget's disease in a 66-year-old man: CT with emboli Note the lytic nature of the tumor and the Pagetian changes

Fig. 9. Spindle cell sarcoma arising from origin of the lateral arch of L5 and extending to the vertebral body and the pedicles, to L4, and to the soft perivertebral tissue. The patient presented with sciatic pain radiating from L5 left. Note the osteocondensing aspect of the tumor. Pulmonary metastasis was present

Fig. 10. Lytic osteosarcoma of D5

a

b

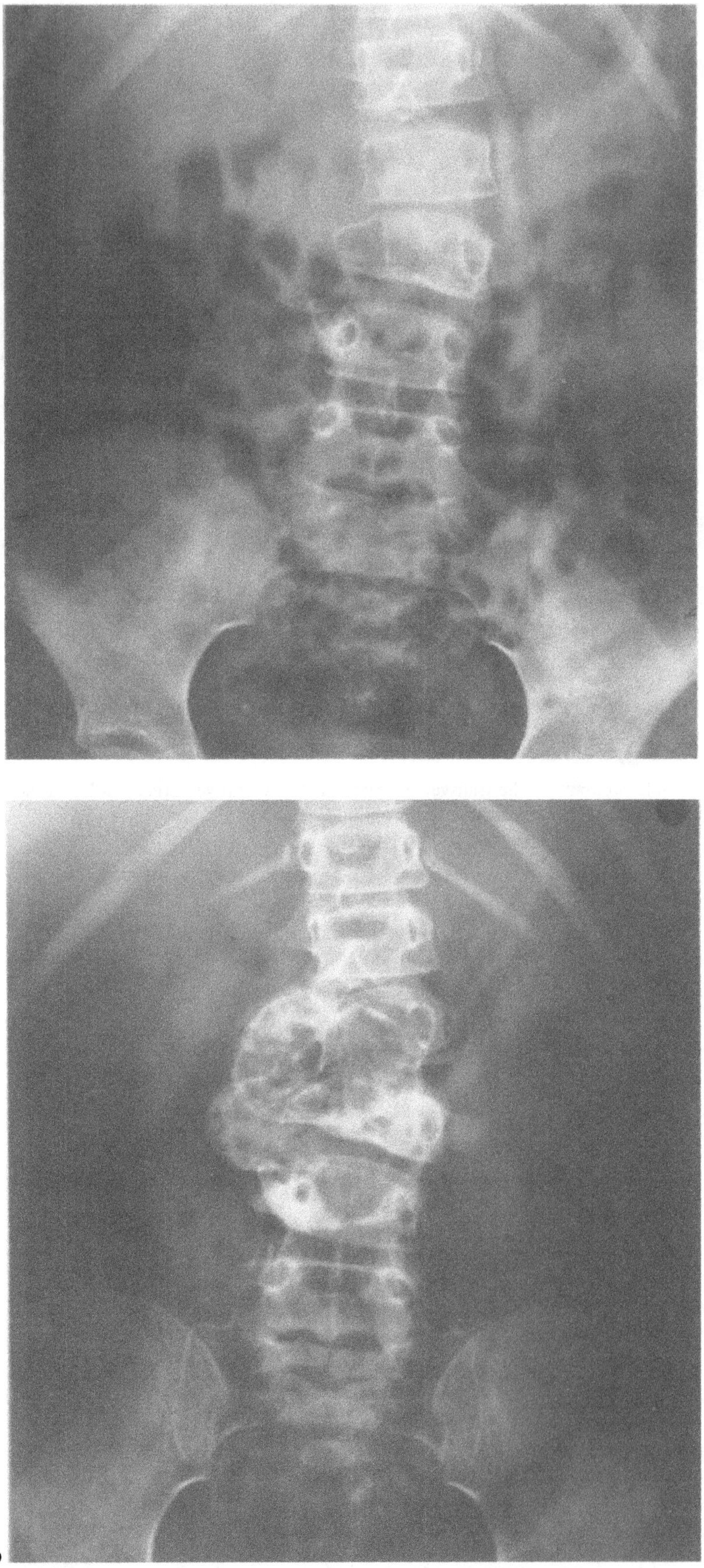

Fig. 12 a, b. Giant cell tumor of the right part of the vertebral body and of the right transverse process of L3. **a** Note appearance with jodgements and absence of invasion of L2 and L4 despite tumor volume; **b** at 1 year later, evident invasion of L2 and L4 and appearance of osteocondensed zones

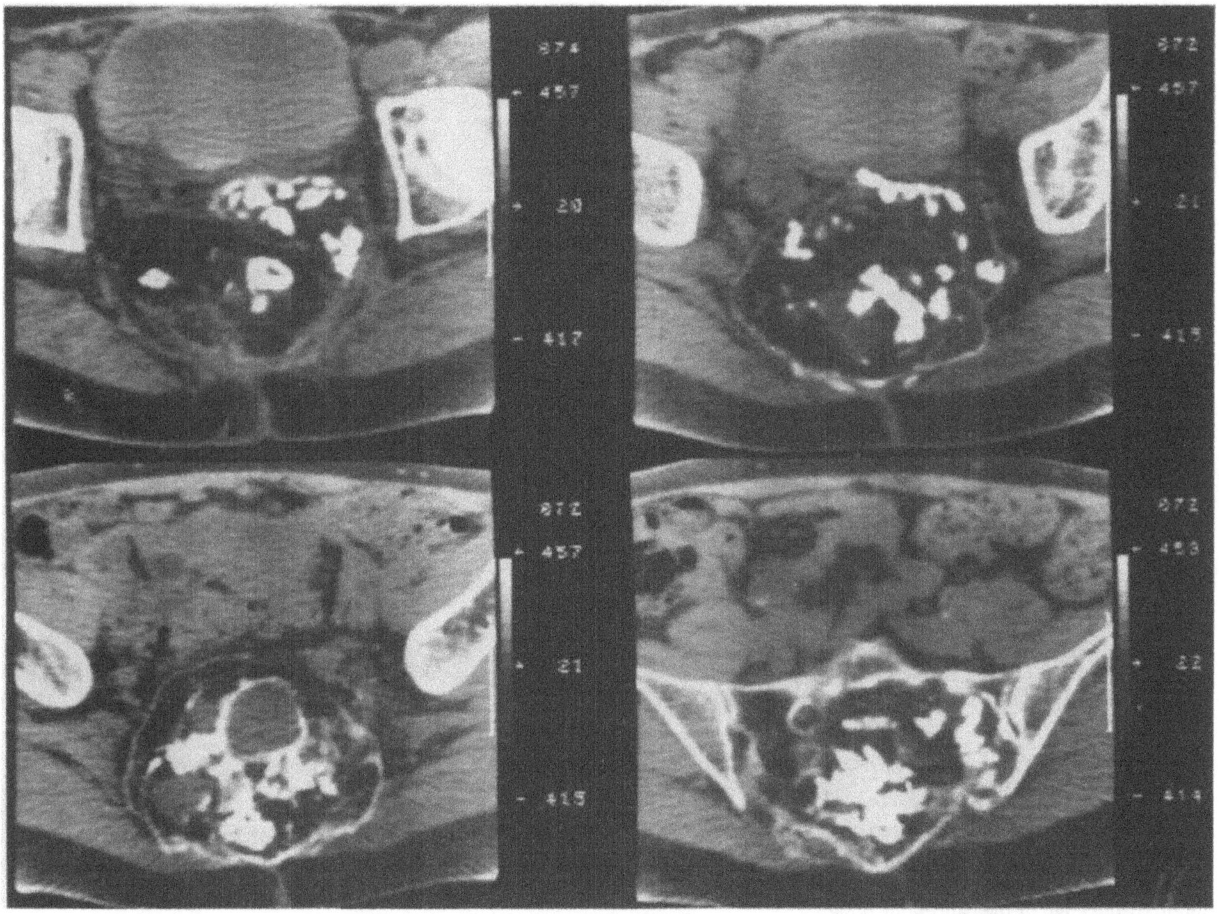

Fig. 13. Status in a 60-year-old woman treated by radiotherapy in 1950 for giant cell sarcoma of the sacrum. No progression in 30 years. Final diagnosis, osteoclastoma

IX. Tumors Originating from the Bone Marrow and Blood Elements

Such tumors are rarely benign, and some cases of xanthomas have been reported.

1. Myeloma and Plasmocytoma

The vertebral column is the most frequent site of multiple myelomas, which account for 10%–15% of primary tumors of the spine. The dorsal level is most often affected, with a high proportion of immediately plurifocal forms. In the majority of cases the tumor originates from the vertebral bodies. These tend to fragment the bone, replacing it with a gelatinous mass, to the point where it overflows the vertebral body limits, most often following a pathologic deformation. We can thus observe paravertebral masses, an extension to the adjacent levels, or compressive syndromes of the marrow and of the cauda equina. Direct extension toward the spinal cord is apparently prevented by the dura mater in the vast majority of cases.

Different groups of lytic forms have also been described:

Cystic areas of thinning, with the appearance of soap bubbles.

Forms simulating senile osteoporosis, with biconcave deformations of the vertebral body, increased disk thickness, and sometimes tiny cortical erosions. The presence of further tumors of this type at other localizations (e.g., cranium and extremities), is a valuable aid to diagnosis.

Sclerosing forms, condensing, with increased trabeculation.

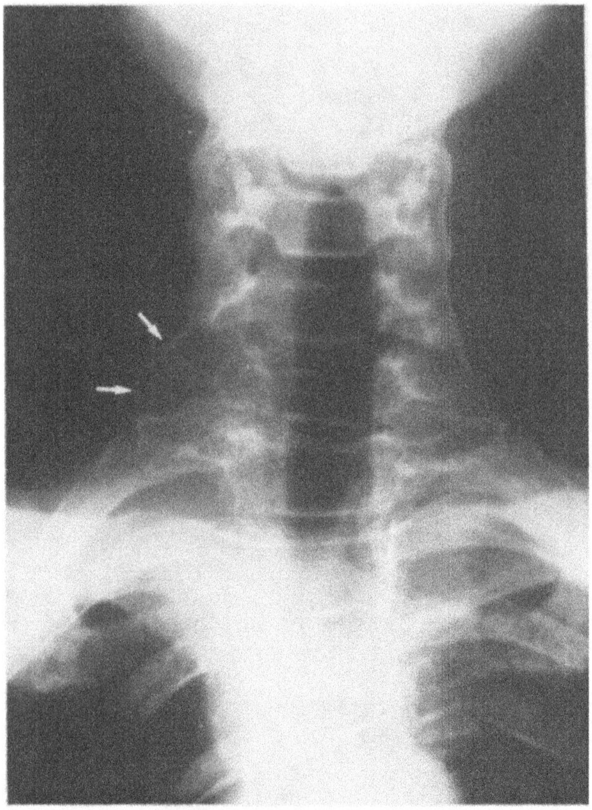

Fig. 14. Myelomatous tumor localized on left lateral mass of C7. Purely lytic appearance. Conservation of a very fine and irregular cortical border, signifying centrifugal growth of the tumor, at the edge of the cancellous bone

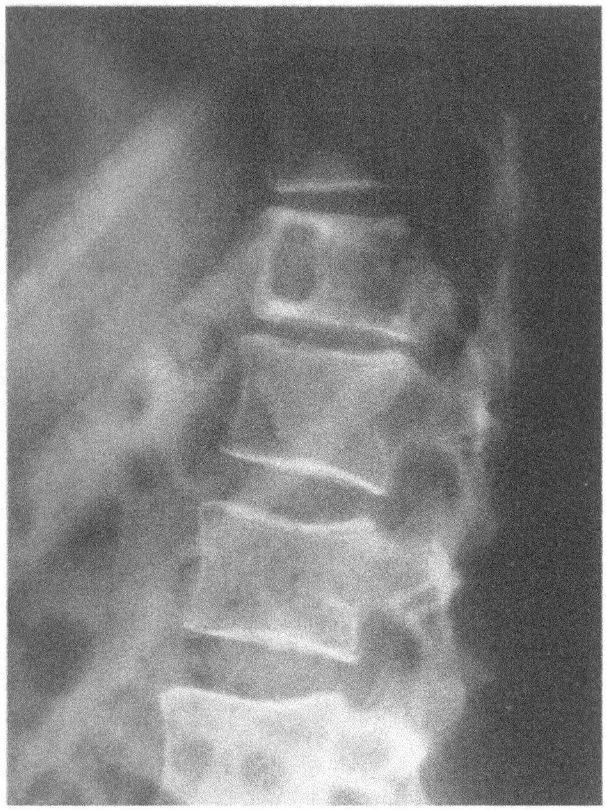

Fig. 15. Myeloma in T11. Note transparent lacuna with scleral borders, anterior and infiltration of the posterior part of the vertebral body of pure lytic type

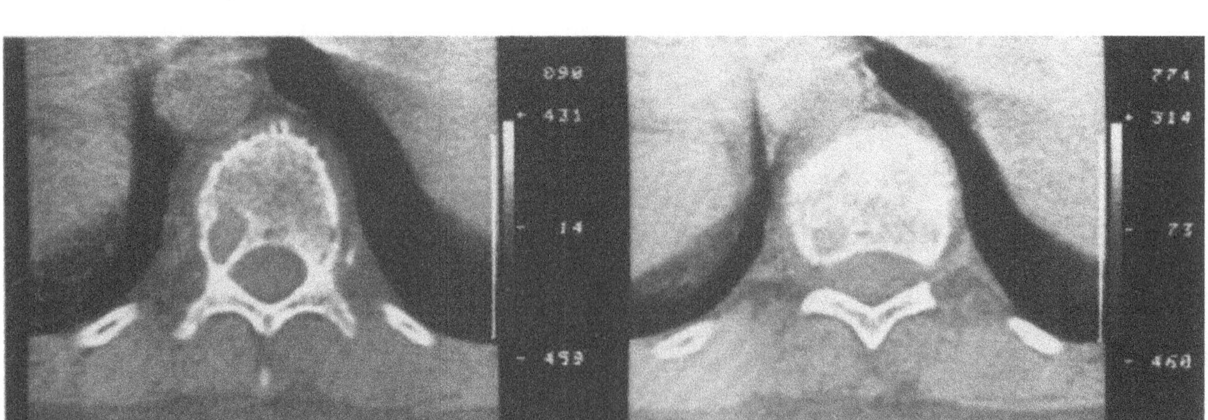

Fig. 16. Incipient myelomatous infiltration of Th10: lytic lacuna representing the fleshy tumor, and thickening of the soft perivertebral tissues

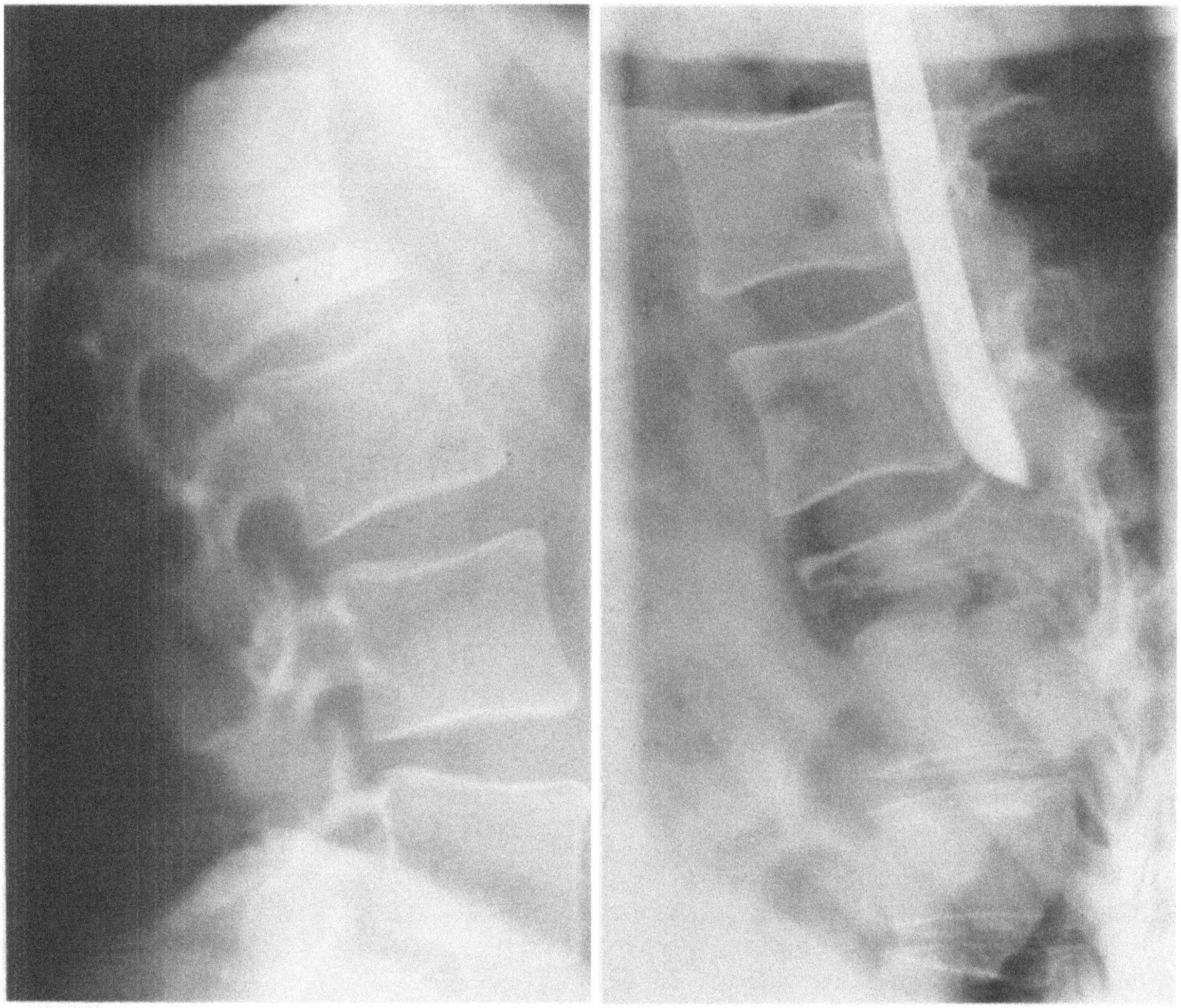

a b

Fig. 17a, b. Man of 48 years presented with lumbago and progressive paraplegia. Examination revealed lytic deformation of L1 by a reticulosarcoma. **a** Lateral view; **b** myelogram (lateral view)

Purely intraspinal forms, epidural, with the clinical picture dominated by neurologic symptoms (Figs. 14–16).

2. Reticulosarcoma, Ewing's Sarcoma

Many writers associate these tumors on the pathological plan, the term Ewing's sarcoma usually being reserved for tumors of the long bones.

They are rapidly expanding lesions, surruounding the dura mater without invading it, and causing major neurologic deficits by compression. They are principally lytic lesions, neoformation of bone reconstructive reaction of the host vertebra or of normal bone being exceptional. Extension to the perivertebral soft tissue and to adjacent levels is observed, as are intracanal (extradural block) and pathologic fractures (Figs. 17–19).

3. Leukemias

Vertebral involvement is encountered as frequently with lymphoid as with myeloid types, and in all age groups. There are various types of lesions:

Infiltration by way of the "sleeve" of the dura mater, the osseous spine being affected by contiguity (scalloping, enlargement of the intervertebral foramen).

Direct osseous infiltration, lytic, with pathologic fractures.

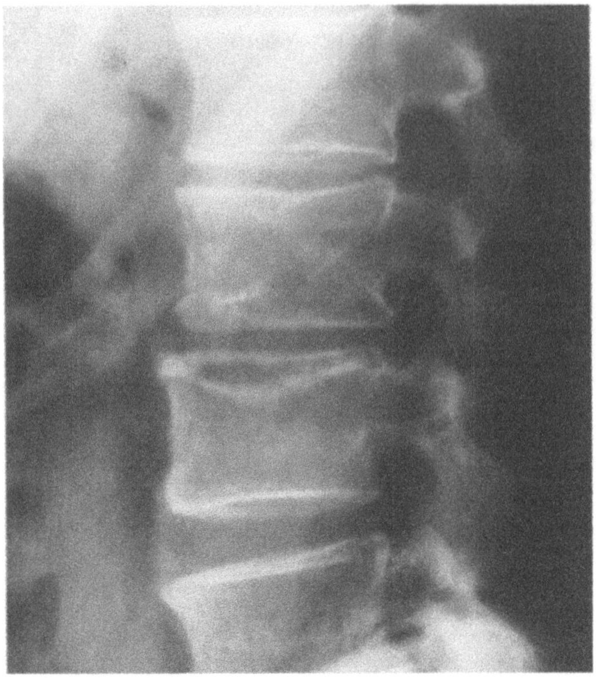

Fig. 18. Man of 66 years old presented with chronic lumbago and was found to have an osteolytic lesion of L2 with pedicular lysis caused by a reticulosarcoma

In children, the appearance of subcortical clear bands at the level of the vertebral plates, similar to those encountered on long bones.

In the chronic forms reactive sclerosis may be seen.

4. Lymphosarcoma

Lymphosarcomas also give rise to lytic vertebral infiltrations, giving a picture identical with that of other spinal sarcomas, but are seen in addition as epidural or paraspinal masses, with invasion of the bone, the meninges, the marrow, or the neural roots themselves.

5. Hodgkin's Disease, Lymphomas

Hodgkin's disease often expands at a less aggressive speed than lymphosarcomas. We would not therefore be astonished to encounter a higher proportion of mixed or blastic forms, varying in severity up to the appearance of "ivory vertebra." In the retroperitoneal forms of lymphomas there are erosions of the anterior vertebral walls (scalloping), and intracanalar invasions by way of the intervertebral foramen or the bloodstream (Figs. 20–23).

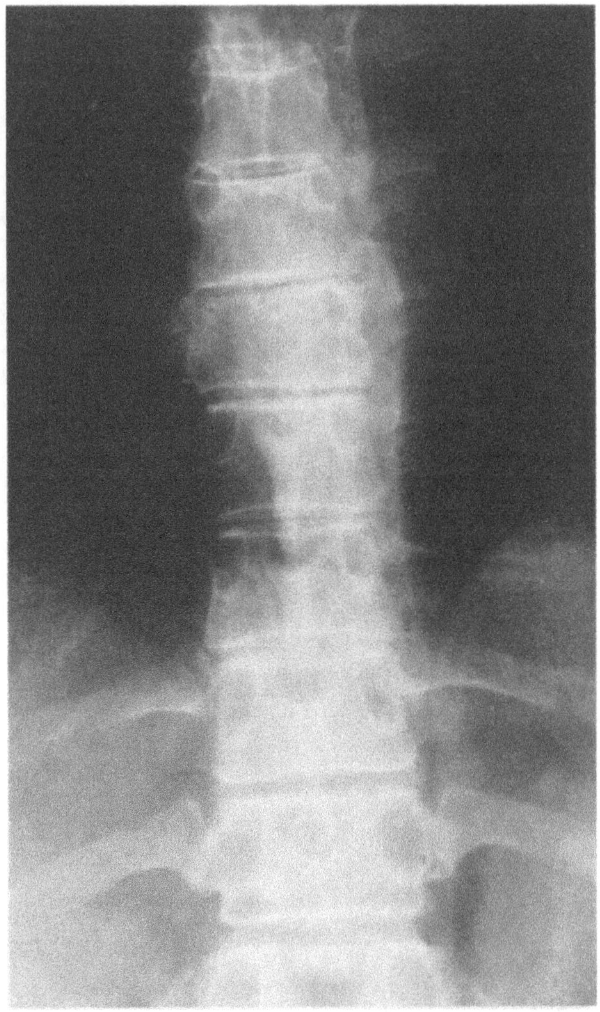

Fig. 19. Woman of 55 years had thoracic pain low in the shoulder girdle and was found to have a lytic lesion of T7 progressing towards total deformation. Skull radiographs were typical for myeloma. Biopsy of D7 revealed a reticulosarcoma (myelosarcoma with plasmocytic differentiation): lytic lesion of T7

6. Myelosclerosis

Myelosclerosis is characterized radiologically by diffuse changes in the trabeculation of the vertebrae without modification of the contours, the density of the osseous stroma being increased to give it a grosser aspect.

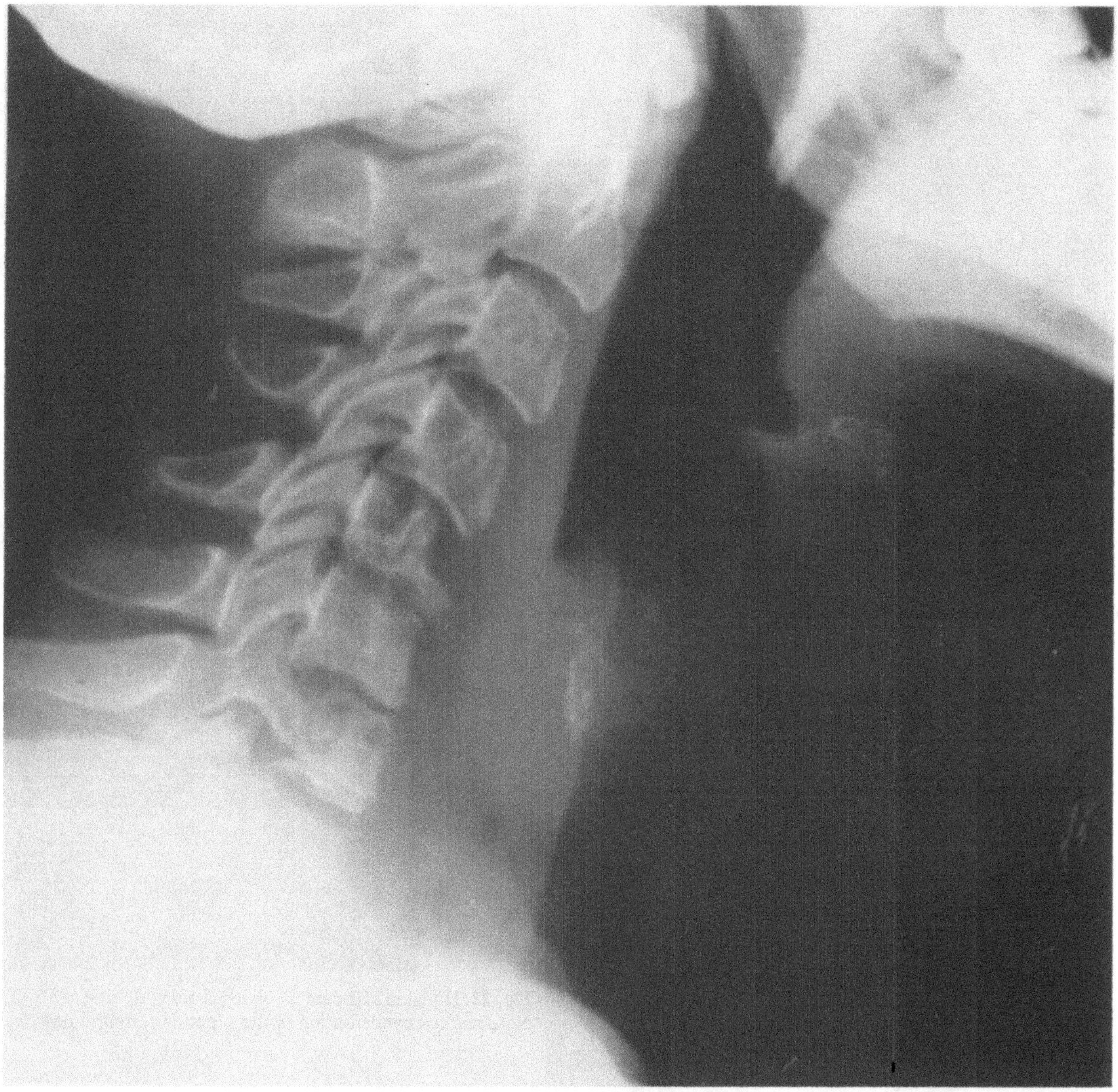

Fig. 20. Hodgkin's disease infiltrating body of C5, essentially lytic

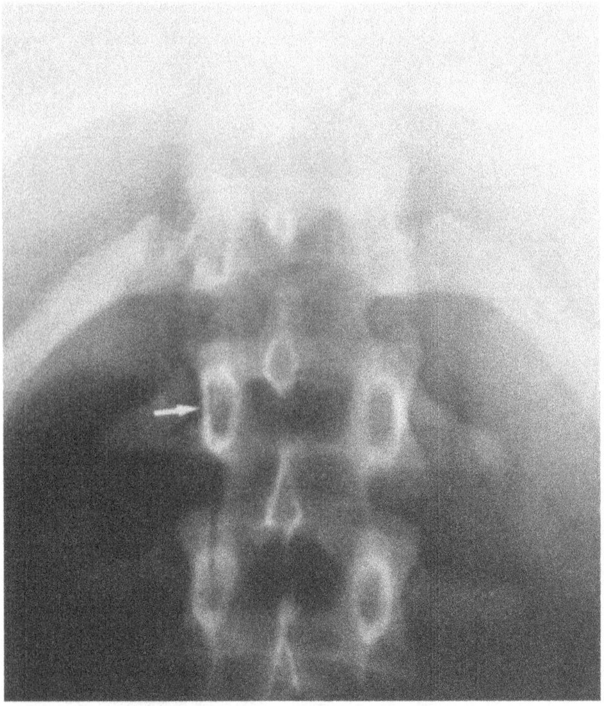

a

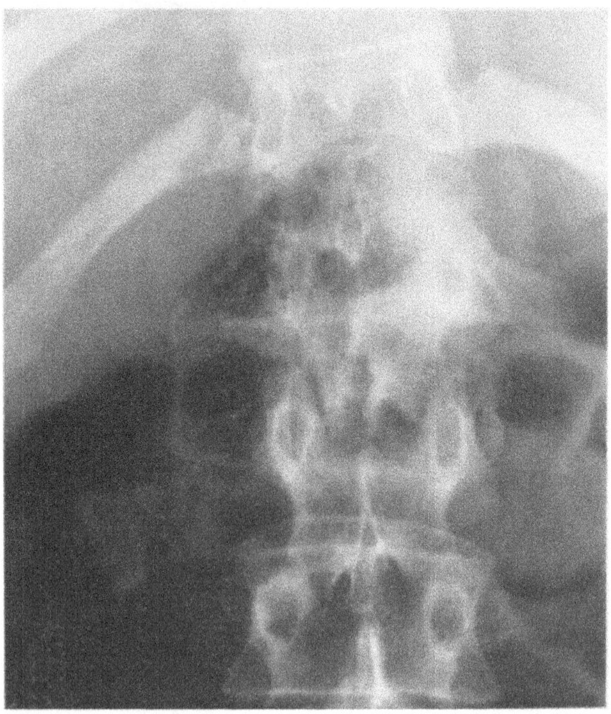

b

Fig. 21. a Hodgkin's disease infiltrating L1, reflected in a moderate trabecular relaxation visible at the right pedicle (*arrow*; **b** the same patient after 1 year; note the mixed nature of the osseous reshaping

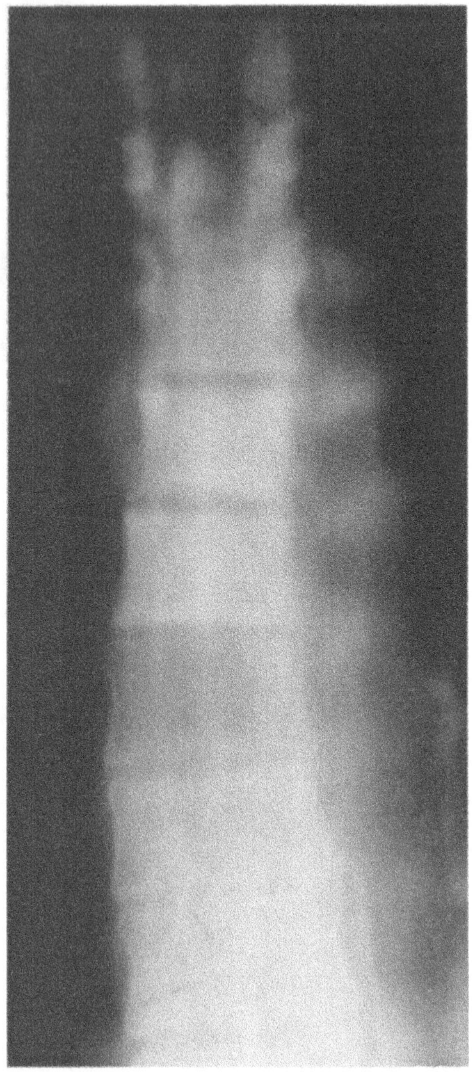

Fig. 22. Hodgkin's disease involving ivory vertebrae at T3–T6. Note marked condensation of the superior vertebral pedicles

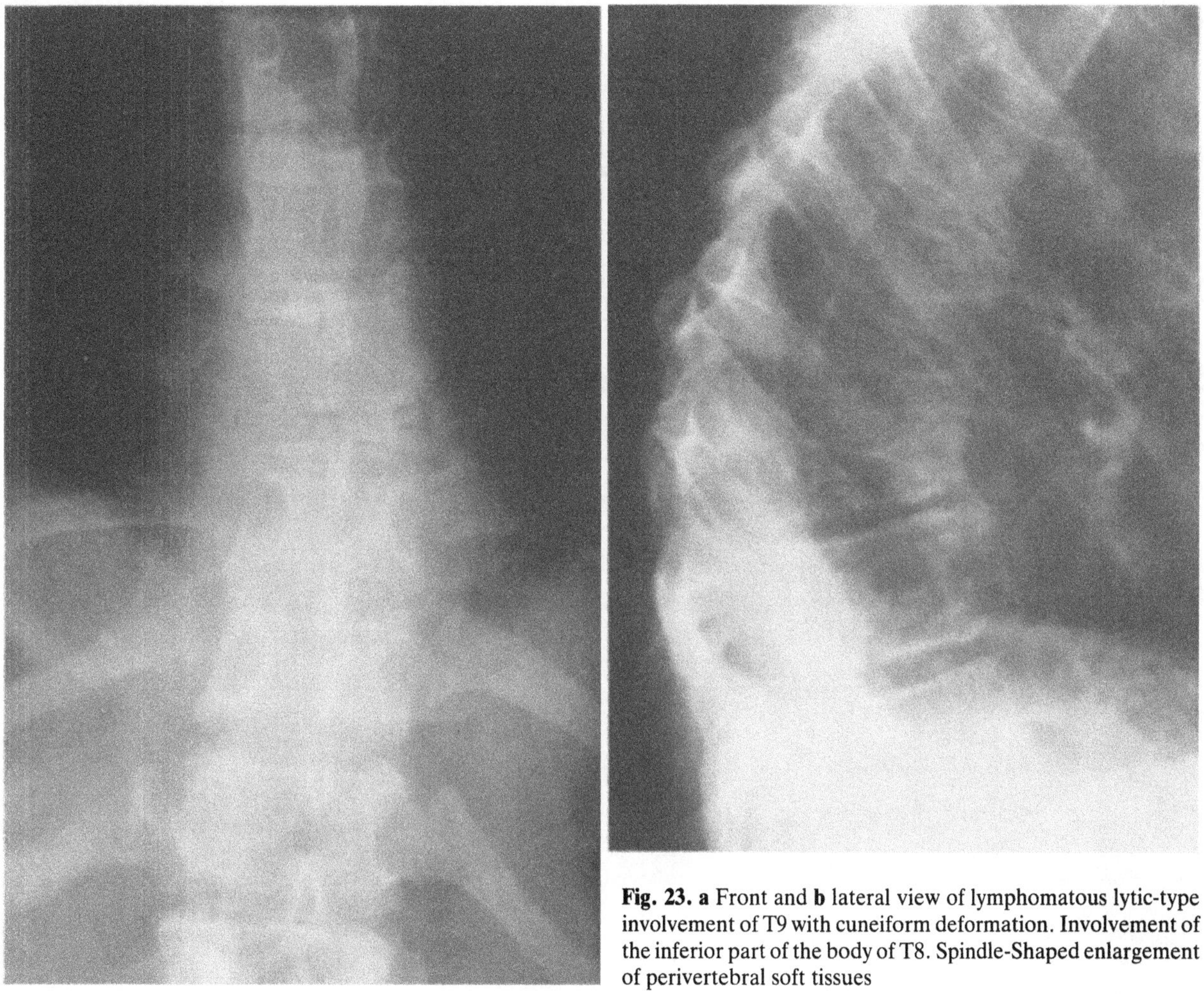

a b

Fig. 23. **a** Front and **b** lateral view of lymphomatous lytic-type involvement of T9 with cuneiform deformation. Involvement of the inferior part of the body of T8. Spindle-Shaped enlargement of perivertebral soft tissues

X. Tumors of Vascular Origin

1. Angiomas

The spine is the most frequent localization of angiomas. Their incidence appeared high in an autopsy series (10%) which included lesions that were not detectable by radiography.

Association with epidural angiomas is not rare. The areas of predilection are the thoracic and lumbar regions, the cervical segment being more rarely affected. Usually isolated, they are revealed as multiple tumors in about 10% of cases, which takes on particular significance in the case of associated neurologic signs, ultimately showing definitely which of the lesions in the clinical picture is the primary one.

The vertebral body is most often affected, showing the typical aspect of a striated (or striped) vertebra, with thinning and spacing of the framework and a global diminution of the osseous density.

The tumor can also extend to the posterior arch, or more rarely, affect this area in isolation. The involvement of the vertebral lamina can lead to stenosis of the canal or of an intervertebral foramen. Deformation of the vertebral body also occurs, in which its walls become convex, giving it a barrel-like appearance.

The majority of these tumors are asymptomatic and are diagnosed fortuitously; they can cause clinical manifestations, in particular painless and progressive paralysis in the event of decompensa-

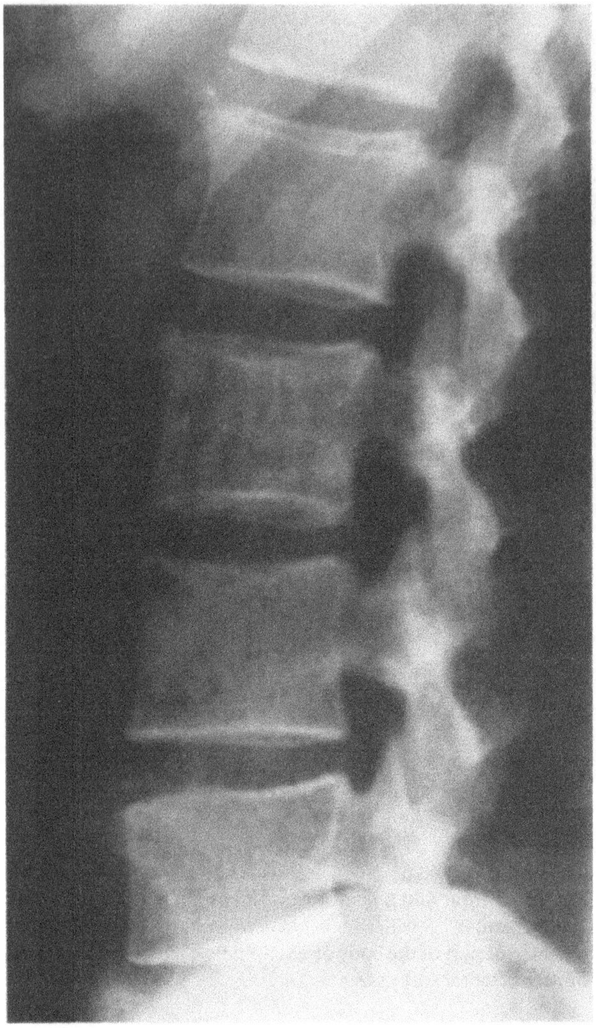

Fig. 24. Angioma of L2

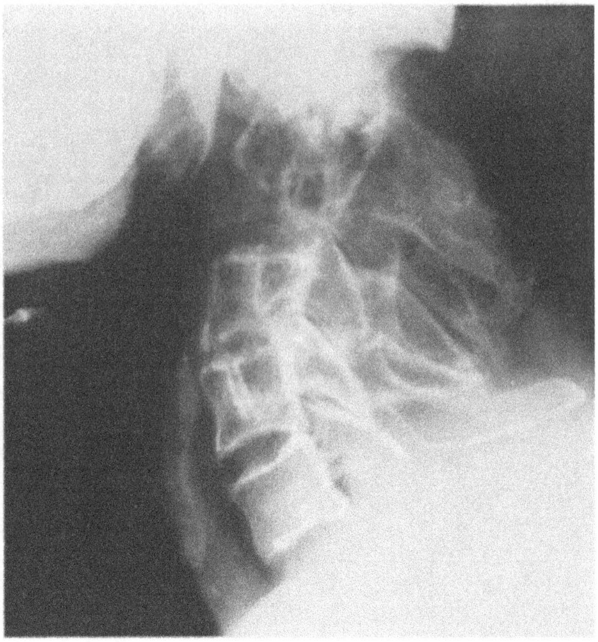

Fig. 25. Cervical angioma of body of C3, purely lytic

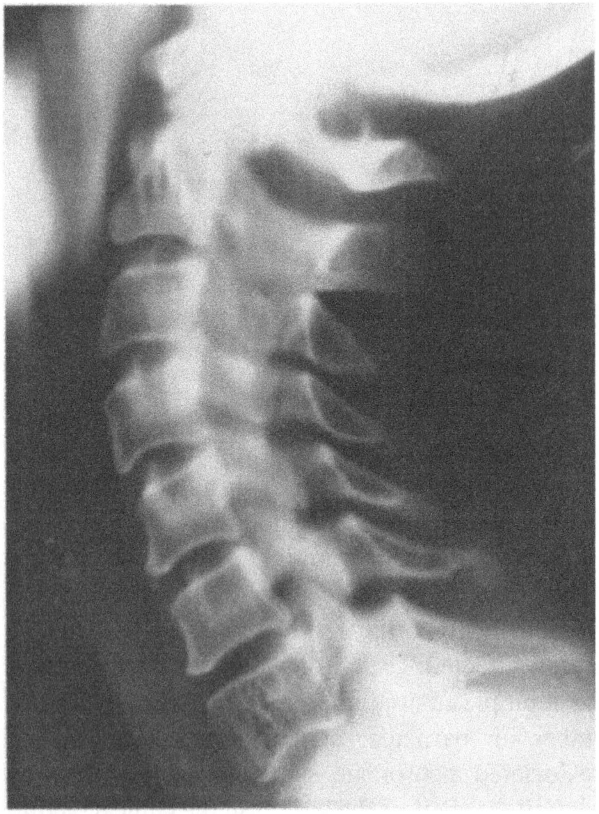

Fig. 26. Angioma of C7

Fig. 27a, b. Angioma of left pedicle and left posterior arch of L1: **a** Standard roentgenogram; **b** tomogram

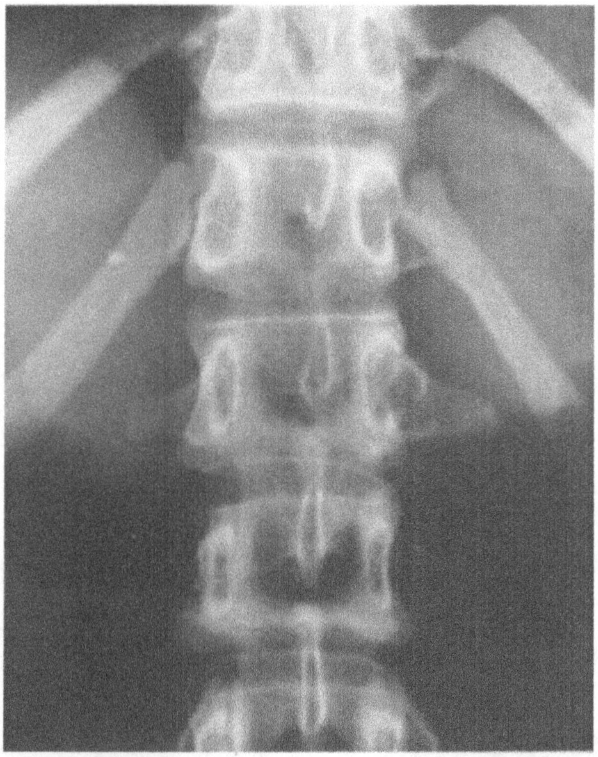

a

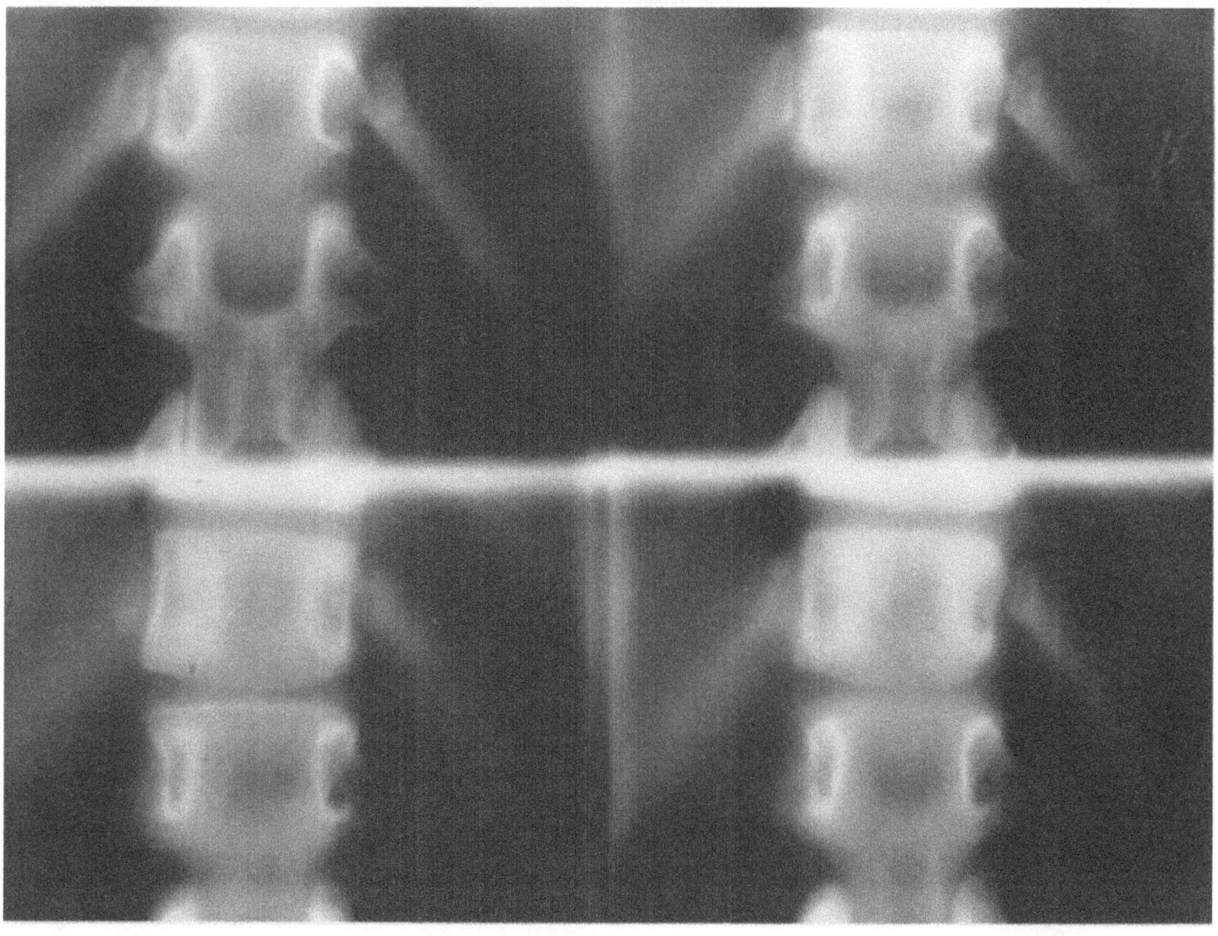

b

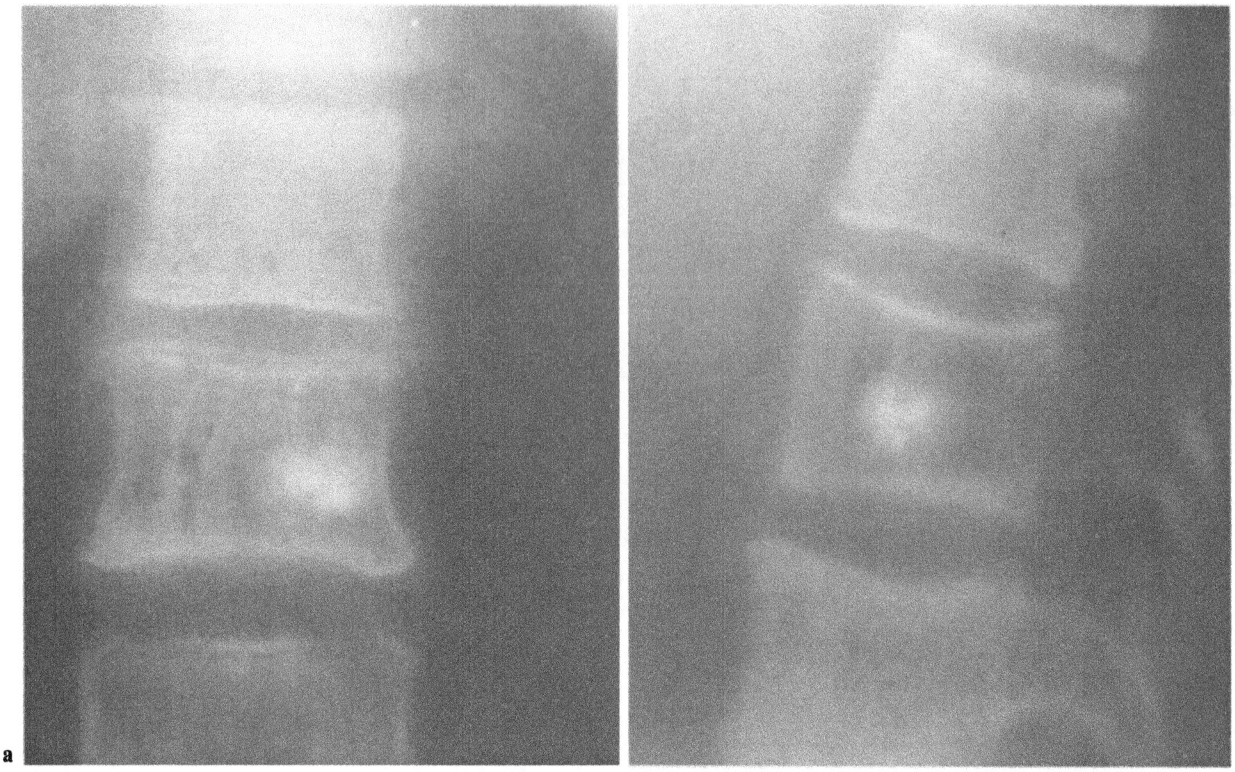

Fig. 28a, b. Angioma of body of L2 with islet of osteocondensation: **a** front-view tomography; **b** lateral-view tomography

Fig. 29 a–c. Pathologic fracture of T12 observed on angioma, posterior compression, no neurologic signs. **a** arteriograph; **b** front-view myelograph; **c** lateral-view myelograph ▷

Fig. 30. Angioma of L1. Axial section shows intracorporeal localization of the lesion: conservation of the cortical content and significant trabecular rearrangements with appearance of more pronounced vertical networks

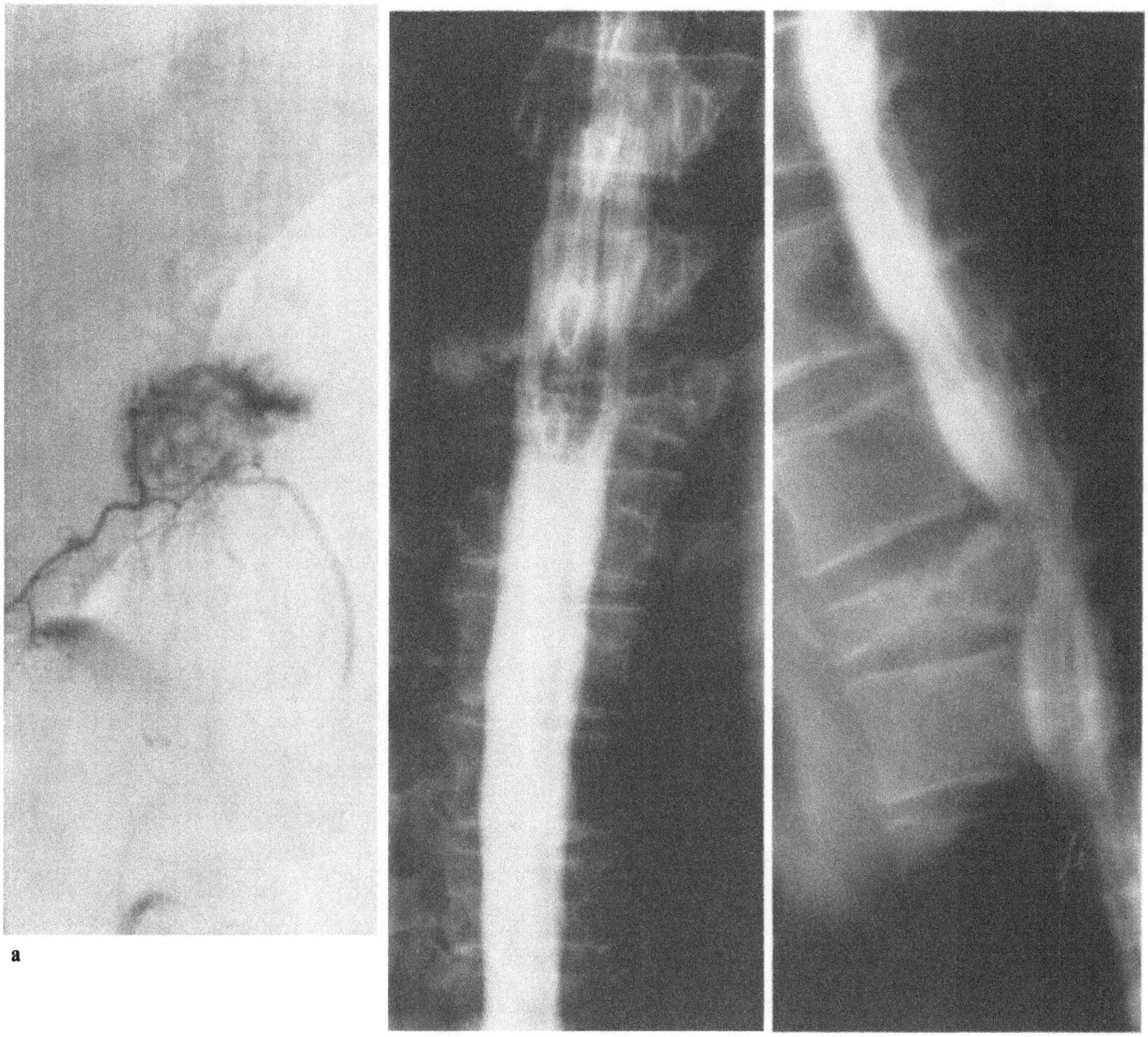

a

Fig. 29 a–c b c

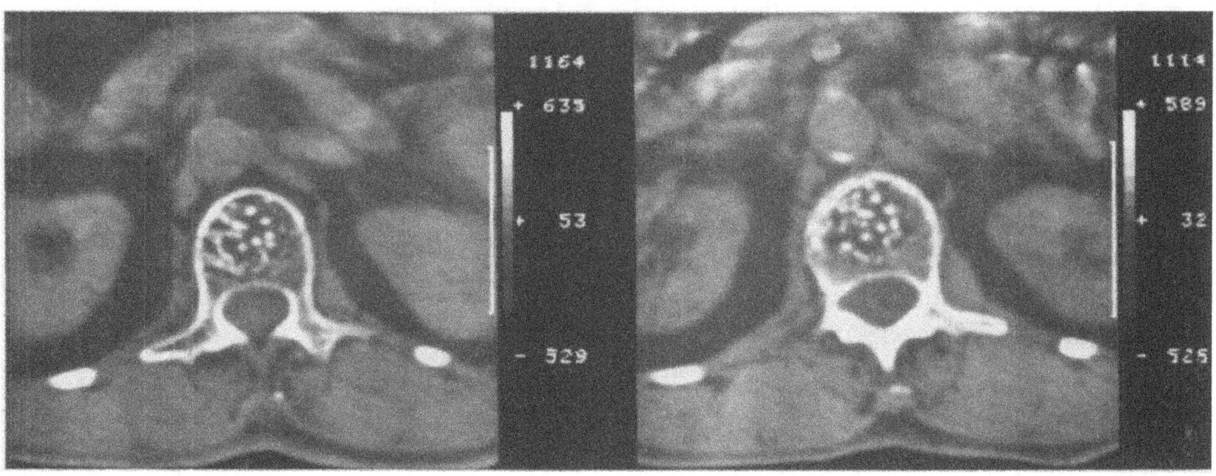

Fig. 30

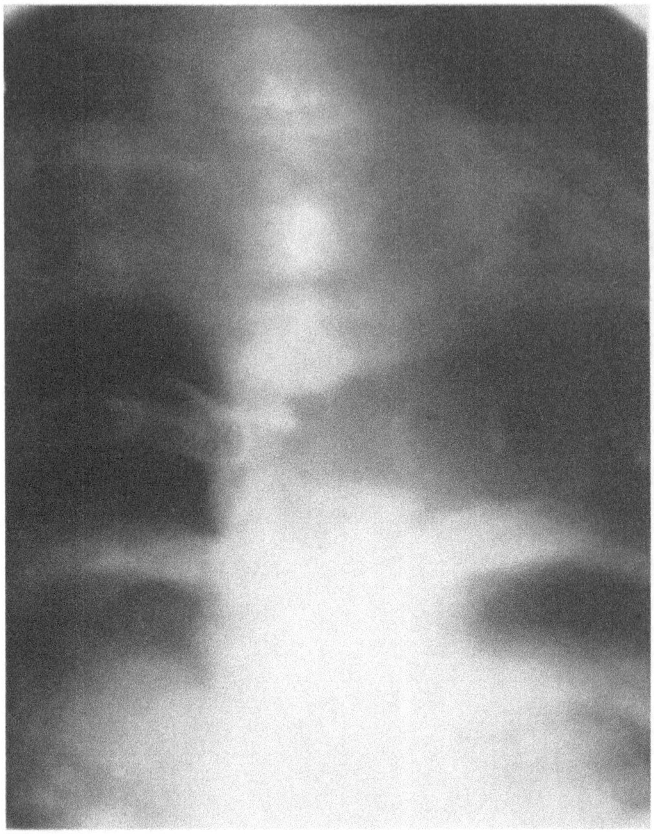

a

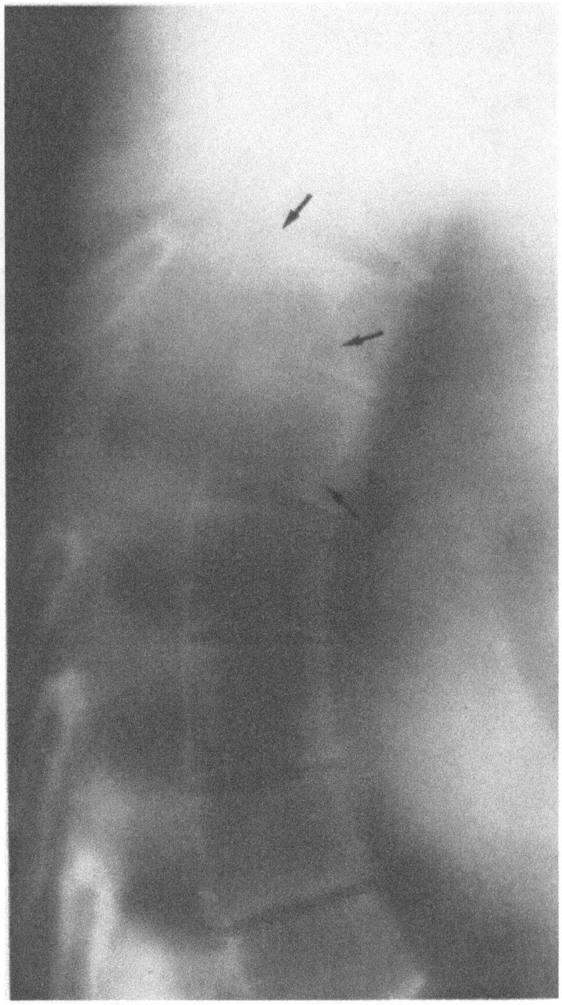

b

Fig. 31 a, b. Hemangiosarcoma involving T3, T4, and the posterior arch of T4 in a woman 48 years of age who presented with a 3-month history of increasingly severe back pain rapidly progressing toward paraplegia. **a** Front view; **b** lateral view

tion. At least a quarter of the mass of the vertebral body must be affected before the typical striated appearance is seen the vertebral end plates and the vertebral walls remaining intact. A concomitant pathologic disk condition can simulate Pott's disease, with the possibility even of spindle-shaped paravertebral soft-tissue swelling. Some lesions can be difficult to differentiate from angiomas: osteogenic sarcomas with a centrovertebral origin (rapidand aggressive behavior); incipient Paget's disease (modified vertebral contours); and osteoporosis (diffuse character of the lesions).

Finally, the pathologic deformation can be present immediately, making identification improbable (Figs. 24–30).

2. Lymphangiomas

Rare in the spine, lymphangiomas are seen as plaques of osseous thinning, sometimes with reconstructive reactions.

3. Cystic Angiomatosis

Cystic angiomas in vertebral sites have the appearance of purely lytic lesions, generally encircled by a border of sclerosis and with no extravertebral extension.

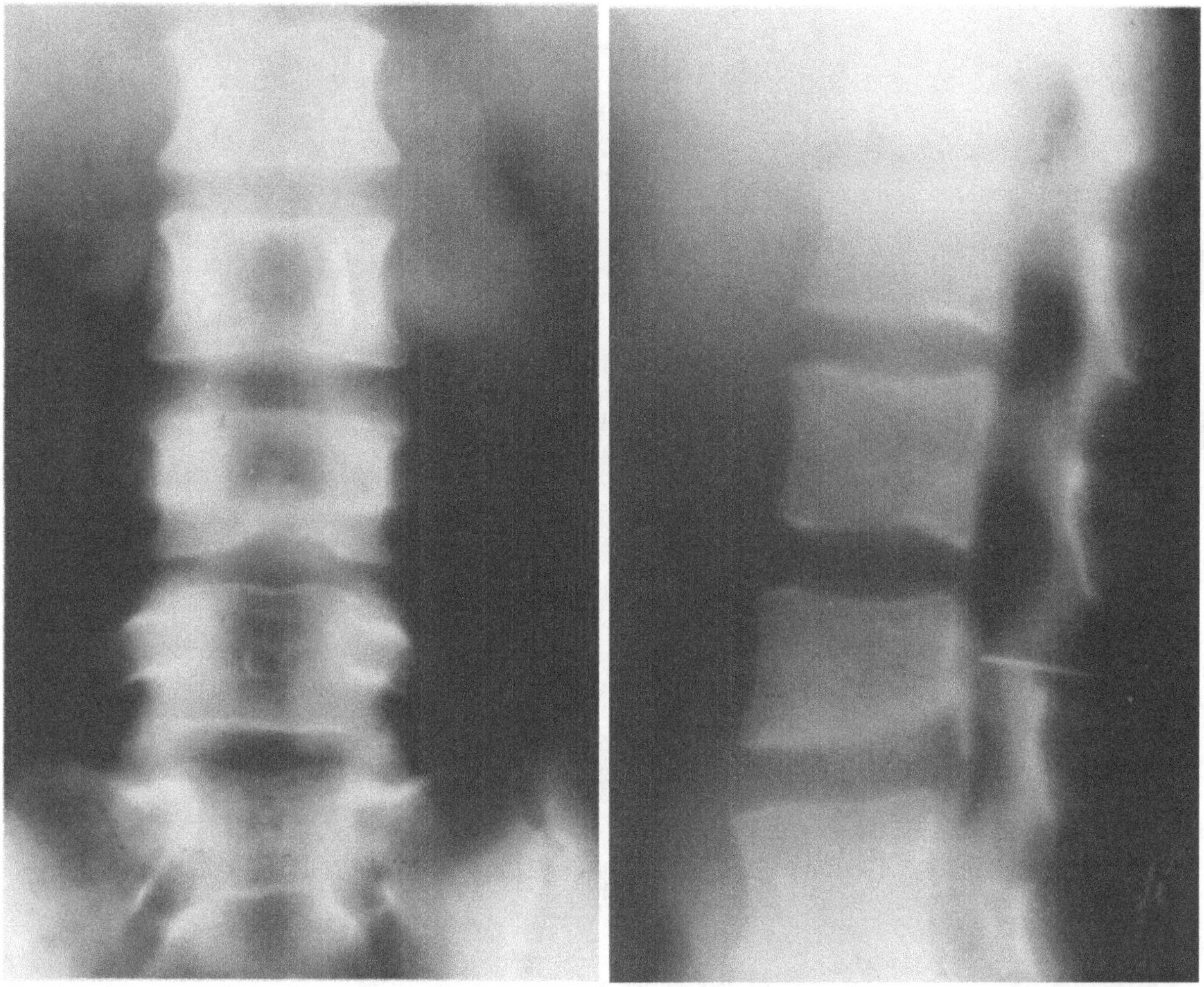

a b

Fig. 32 a, b. A man 38 years old presented with badly defined lumbago with no neurologic deficit. Chordoma was found occupying the posterior inferior part of L4, eroding the inferior plate and displacing the posterior inferior wall backward. **a** Front view; **b** lateral view

4. Hemangiosarcomas

Of lytic predominance, a hemangiosarcoma can involve an entire vertebra or only a part of it; intracanalar extension perivertebrally or toward adjacent levels is frequent. The differential diagnosis must consider other sarcomatous tumors and metastatic lesions but is often impossible (Fig. 31).

5. Chordomas

Derived from notochord remnants, chordomas represent 15%–20% of primary vertebral tumors. The preferred sites are the clivus and the base of the cranium, and the lumbosacral junction (sphenoid localizations are not discussed here).

These are soft tumors, rounded and locally invasive, although metastases appear in the late stages. They form lytic lesions with regular contours, often spreading over seyeral vertebral levels, and can destroy the disk. Calcic debris can be seen at the center of the tumor (the most typical image is that of destruction of many adjacent vertebral bodies with involvement of the disk spaces). Posterior extension can bring on myelocompressive syndromes, while anterior extension can cause backward displacement of the prevertebral or pelvic structures (The treatment is usually pallative, consisting in curettage and radiotherapy. The lesion is always fatal in the medium or long term (Figs. 32–37).

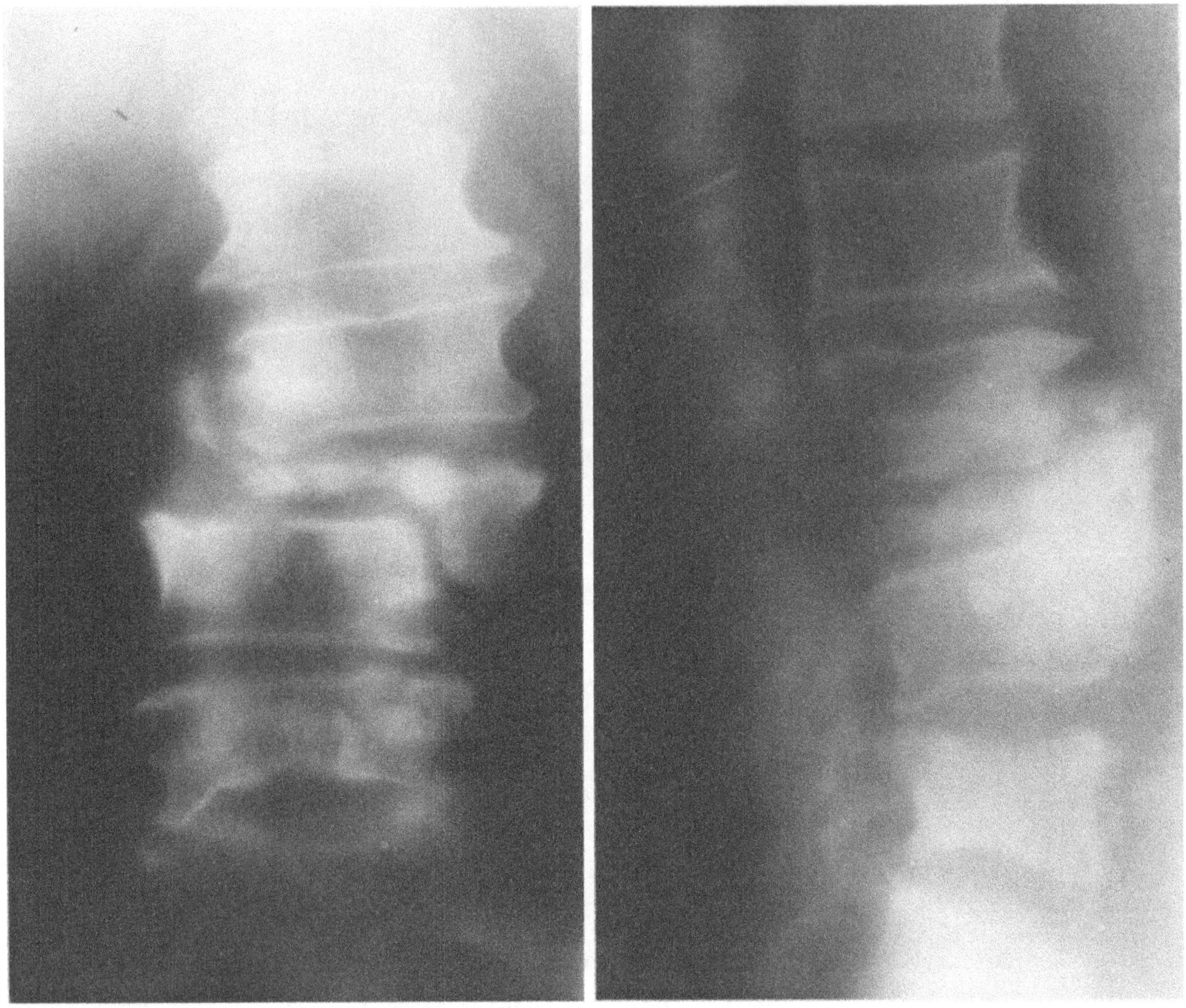

a b

Fig. 33 a, b. Chordoma of L3 with pathologic deformation and anterior protusion. **a** Front view; **b** lateral view

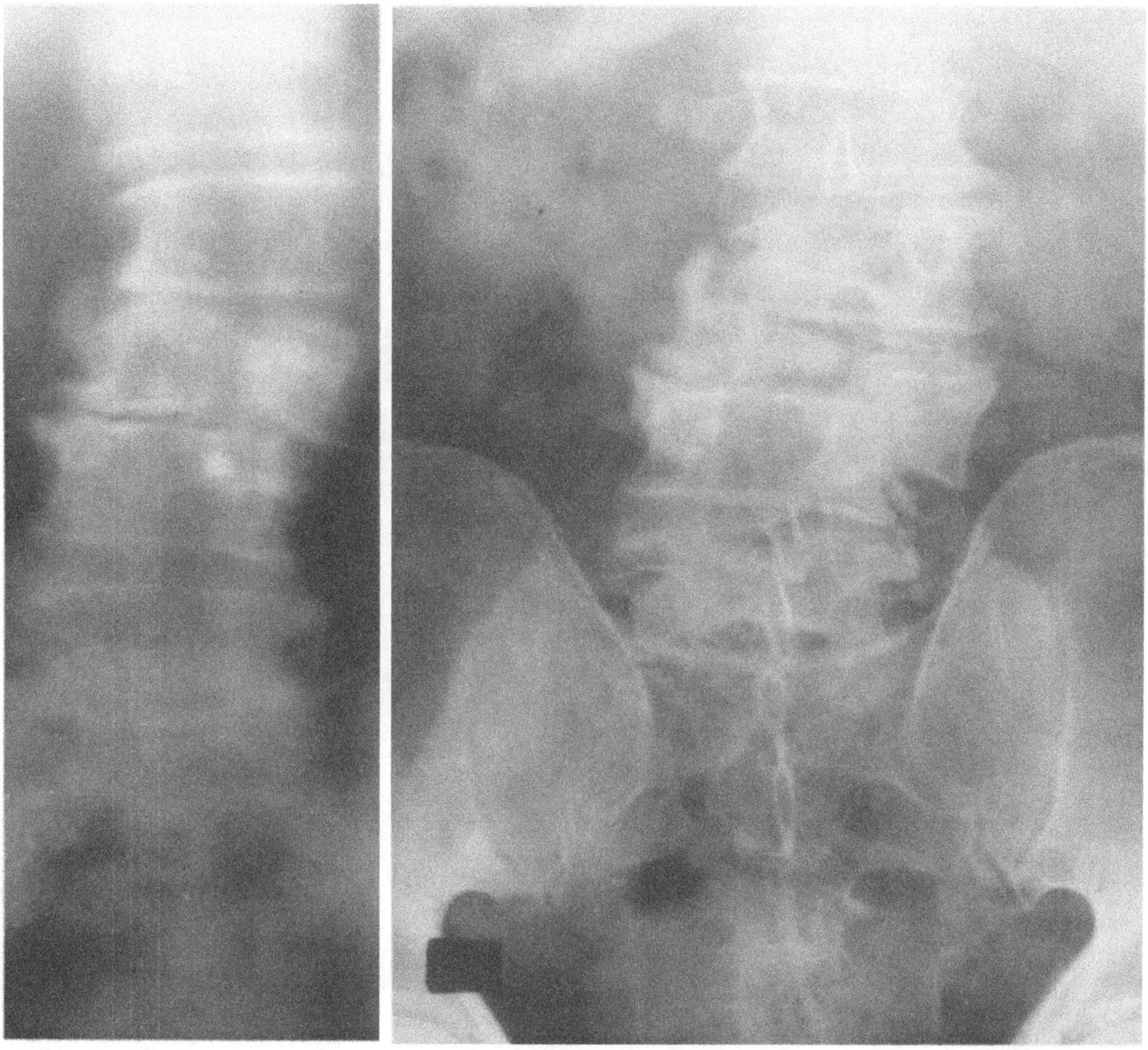

a b

Fig. 34. a Chordoma of L3, also invading the superior half of the body of L4, in a man of 70 years. **b** Same tumor 2 years later

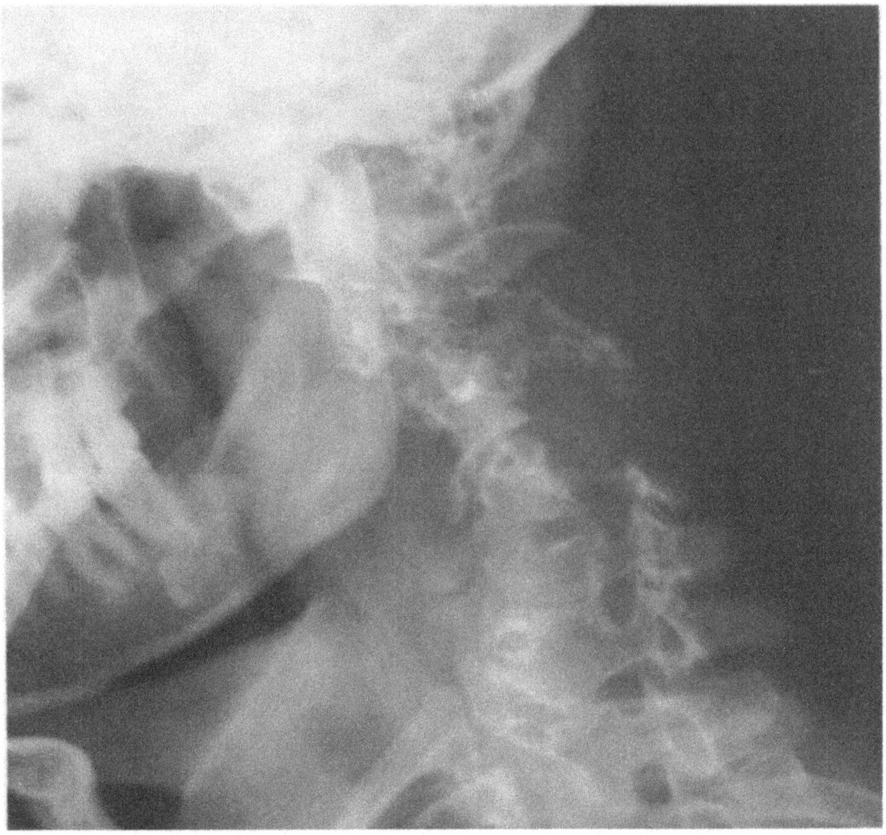

Fig. 35

Fig. 36 a–d ▽

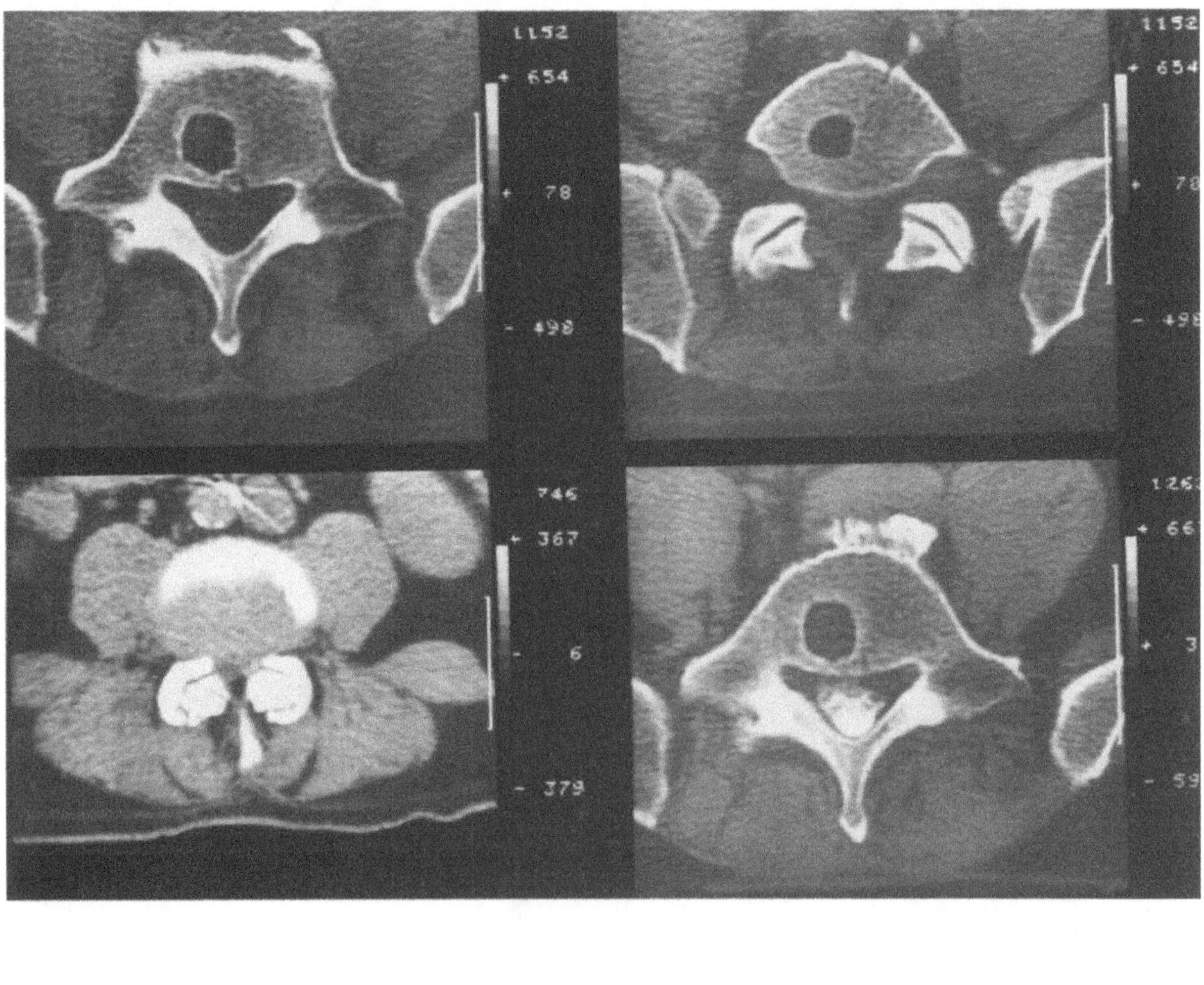

b c a d

◁ **Fig. 35.** Chordoma of C5 with posterior development involving the whole of the posterior arch and eroding the articular processes of C4 and C6

Fig. 36. a Narrow lumbar canal (arthrotic) at L3, L4 and disk protrusion; **b–d** well-circumscribed lytic lesion of body of L5, revealed as chordoma by biopsy

Fig. 37. a Lysis of sacrum at S2 (coccyx) by a solid presacral formation protuding in to the pelvis and revealed as a sacrococcygeal chordoma; **b** computed tomography
▽

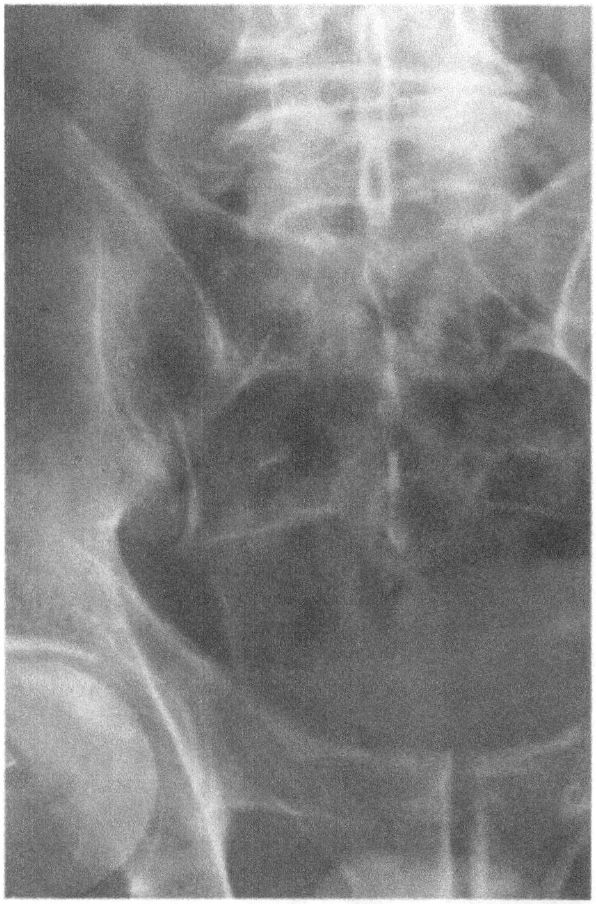

a

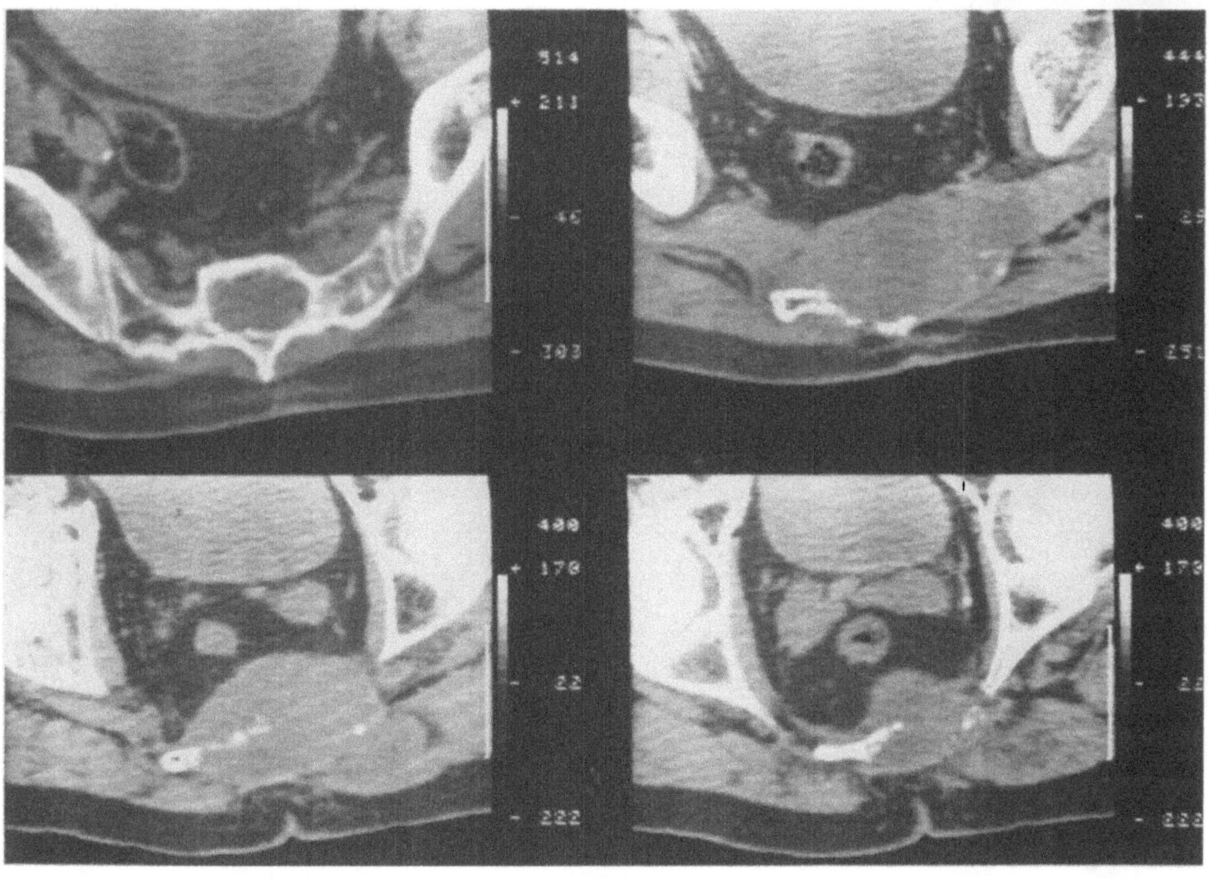

b

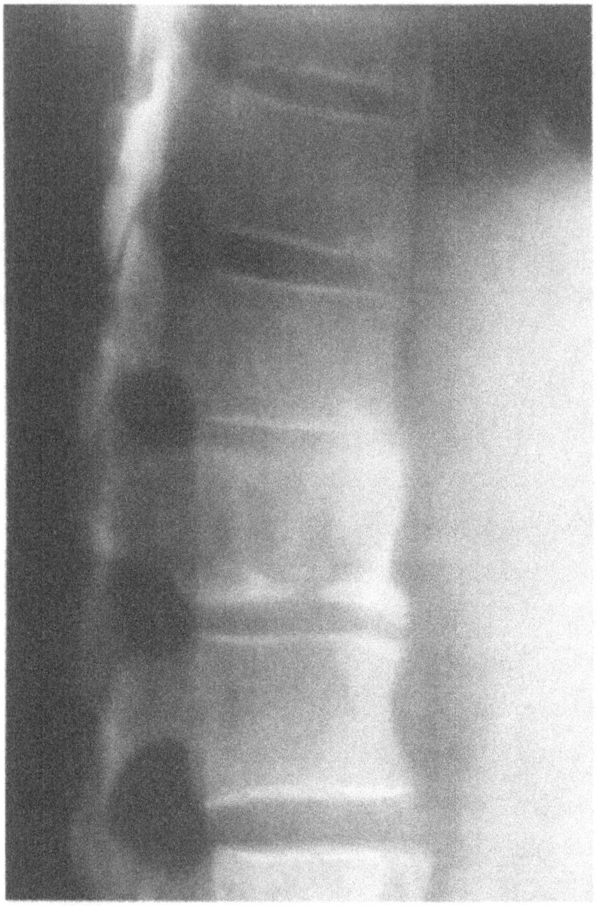

Fig. 38. Aneurysmal cyst of body of T12. Note the well-circumscribed appearance of the lesion, which extends just to the limits of the vertebral body

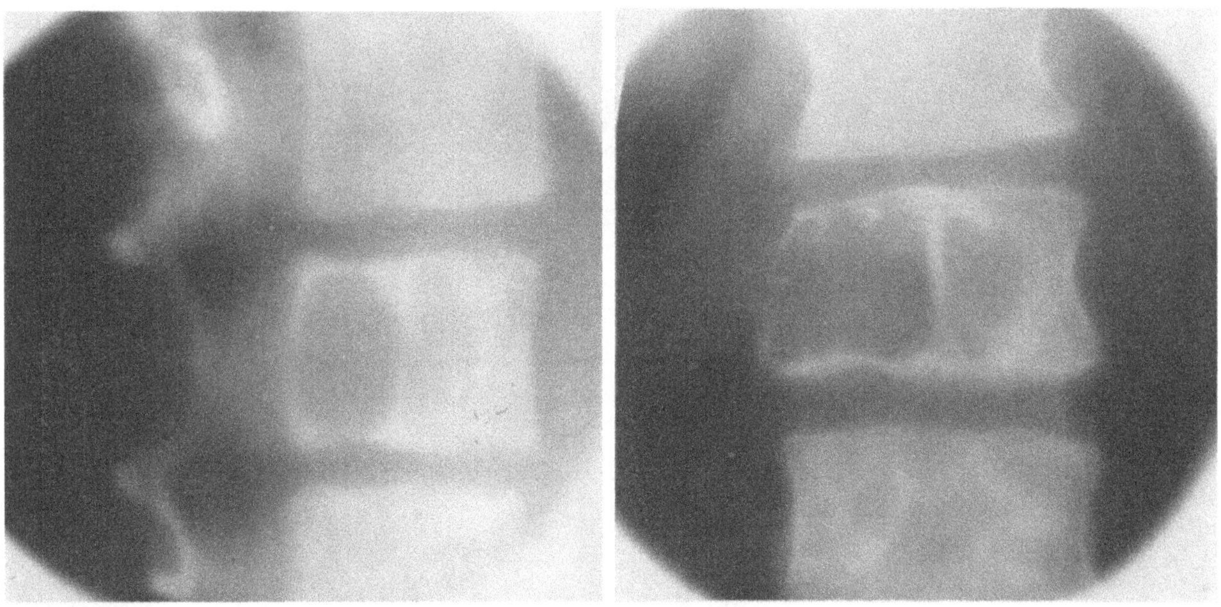

Fig. 39. Aneurysmal cyst of the right part of body of L2 and of right pedicle

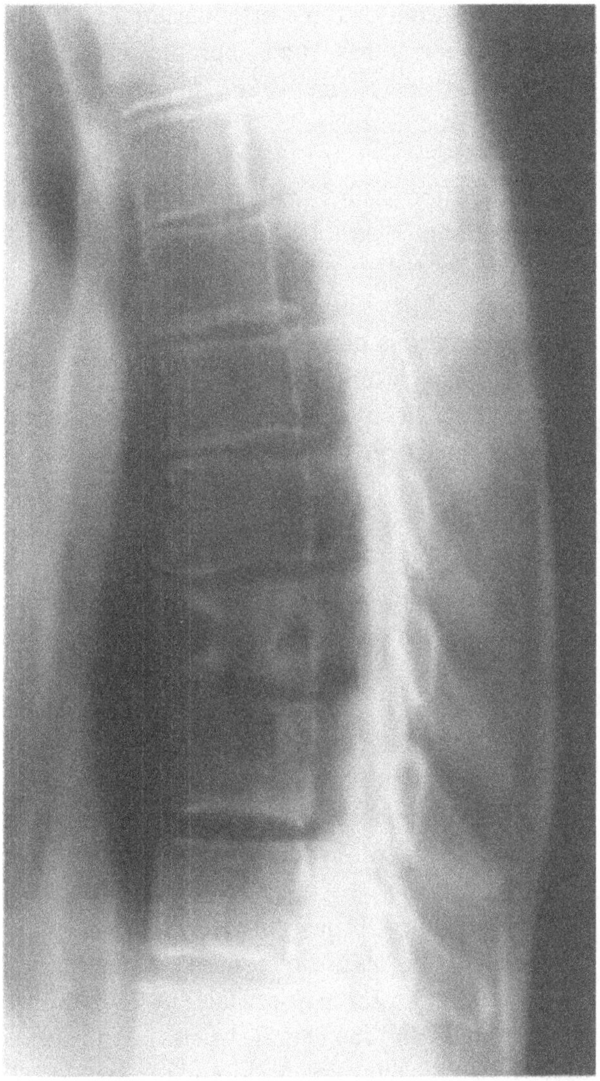

Fig. 40. Aneurysmal cyst of body of T8

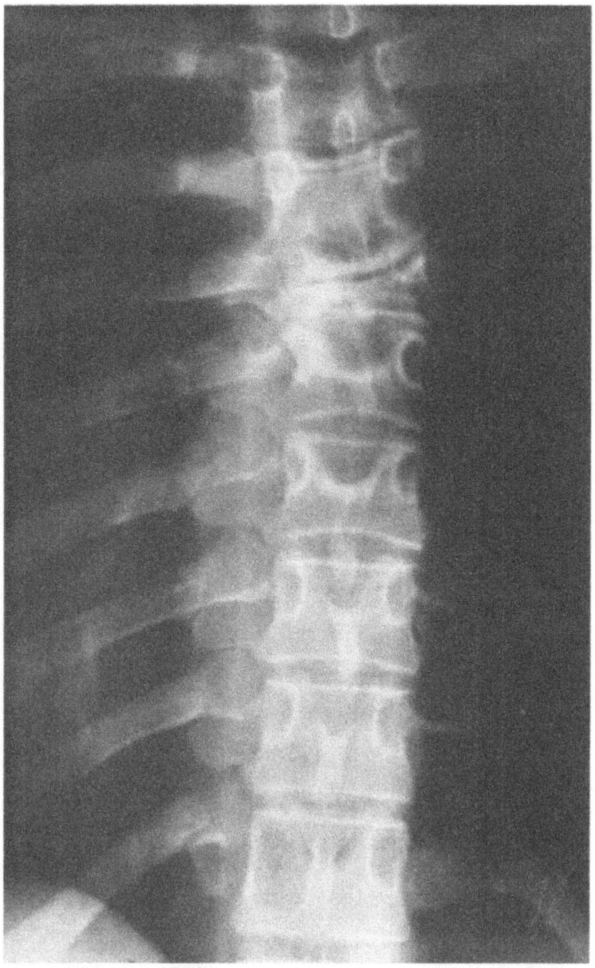

Fig. 41. Woman of 20 years with paraplegia following childbirth. Deformation of T4, lesions also present at T10 and at the cranial vault

C. Pseudo- or Paratumoral Lesions

I. Aneurysmal Cyst

Vertebral localization of aneurysmal cysts is frequent, the most frequent site according to Lichtenstein; the patients are young, mainly in the first 2 decades (male predominance in age group 10–30 years). The cervical and thoracic regions are the most often attacked and the lesion generally occurs in isolation and is localized to a single vertebra. It is always encapsulated, but it can push back the vertebral cortex towards the outside, making it convex with an eggshell appearance, particularly at the level of the neural arch. Erosion of the adjacent vertebra and vertebral deformations are also encountered.

Osseous septa endings divide this tumor into lobules, which are often radiologically visible, but this is more unusual in the spine than in other localizations (Figs. 38–40).

II. Eosinophilic Granuloma

Considered a type of histiocytosis X, eosinophilic granuloma affects mainly individuals under 20 years of age. In about 50 % of cases such tumors are also present at other localizations, particularly in the flat bones. In the early stage it appears as well — defined intraosseous lacunae, but the at which diagnosis is possible is that of vertebral deformations, cuneiform or pebble — shaped, which are highly suggestive in a child. The horizontal diameter of the vertebral body is increased. The clinical picture is characterized by pain, sometimes with radicular or medullary compression, or gibbosity (Fig. 41).

D. Conclusion

Witn the exception of certain entities that have a more characteristic appearance when they arise in their typical form, the diagnosis of tumorous lesions of the vertebral column is often difficult when only radiologic information is available.

The tumors that do frequently present in a distinctive way enclude osteoid osteoma, osteoblastoma, vertebral angioma, some forms of chondroma, and eosinophilic granulomas; their appearance must be considered with reference to the clinical presentation and the age of the patients.

It must be noted that some tumors are polymorphic, in particular the osteogenic sarcomas and the different types of sarcomatous lesions affecting the spine, while on the other hand a similar picture: mixed or lytic movements, extension to the soft tissue or to the adjacent levels, pathologic deformations, can often be caused by any of a number of tumor types. Again, the differential diagnosis must take account of the other lytic lesions that can give rise to the same picture: osteoblastomas, angiomas, plasmocytomas, and multiple myelomas, Hodgkin's disease, metastasis in general, and osteoporotic deformations. The different courses following discovery of the tumor often therefore reflect the impossibility of diagnosing the nature of the tumor (and even of differentiating between a benign and a malignant nature).

Invasion of the soft perivertebral tissue is common to numerous tumorous lesions and to osteomyelitis, and vertebral sclerosis can be encountered in the majority of tumorous syndromes at the center of the lesion, even when diffuse peripherial or distant reactions are present and vary in their degree of homogeneity, as in the case of leukemias, lymphomas, and Pott's disease.

The radiologist's task will therefore be difficult unless all clinical data can be considered together with the radiographic information, especially if the diagnosis and an estimate of the prognosis are anxiously awaited, the latter not always depending on whether or not the tumor malignant. The localization and the sometimes dramatic neurologic consequences are also of primary importance for the patients.

Even though CT has not bed to advances in diagnosis of the nature of tumors, it has proved irreplaceable insofar as it reveals the relation between tumors and the neural structures and shows up lesional mechanisms, besides allowing a check on extension toward the soft tissue in particular.

Spinal Cord Tumors

D. Baleriaux

A. Introduction

Spinal cord tumors are uncommon lesions: according to Rubinstein (26) they account for 15% of all primary tumors of the central nervous system and its sheath elements.

Intramedullary neoplasms are usually slow growing, giving rise to very gradually progressing clinical symptoms of insidious onset [1, 26]. Bony lesions are not always associated with spinal tumors, being caused by excessive intraspinal pressure and arising only after a protracted course in young patients (onset of disease before the age of 30 years). As the normal spinal cord occupies a maximum of half the canalar lumen — at any level of the spinal canal — clinical signs due to total obstruction of the spinal canal can be expected not to appear until after a long period of clinical evolution.

So far, the neuroradiologic procedures necessary for adequate visualization of spinal tumors are difficult and traumatic [2, 4, 5, 11, 17, 25]. Moreover, spinal neoplasms have to be large enough, deform the medullary shape substantially, or alter the medullary shadow in a spectacular way to be detected by "conventional" radiologic procedures [7, 10, 12, 13]. As spinal cord tumors are difficult to detect and observe by means of invasive radiologic examination alone, their natural history is not very well known. Magnetic resonance imaging [22] has recently become available; this offers a totally atraumatic method of studying the spinal cord for the first time. Especially with the aid of surface coils, the intracanalar content can be displayed with anatomic and unmatched precision. This new diagnostic technique will allow earlier detection and improved investigation of intramedullary tumors, and a better understanding of their physiology [16, 18, 21, 23, 30].

B. Radiologic Signs of Spinal Cord Tumors

Following the normal succession of the various radiologic procedures available, the general radiologic signs these procedures can reveal are first discussed.

I. Plain Films of the Spine — Conventional Tomography

It must be stressed that totally normal plain film examinations have been observed in cases of spinal cord tumors. If present, plain film abnormalities will be produced by chronically raised intracanalar pressure: (a) eroded vertebral pedicles, usually bilateral and symmetrical, present in more than one segment; (b) progressive enlargement of the anteroposterior diameter of the bony canal; (c) scalloping of the posterior wall of the vertebral bodies, again seen in several segments. These findings are most frequently associated with ependymomas of the filum terminale and cauda equina and less frequently with astrocytomas or more malignant gliomas, although these combinations are sometimes observed, especially in younger patients.

Calcification is not seen in medullary tumors, and if it is present, extramedullary tumors such as meningioma and, though less frequent, neuromas must be suspected.

Conventional tomography may be very helpful in giving better delineation of bony changes: nevertheless, if the plain film demonstrates signs highly suggestive of spinal cord tumor it is advisable to check these findings by computed tomography (CT). Scoliosis or kyphoscoliosis may also be found associated with spinal cord tumors.

In conclusion, plain film abnormalities are inconstant, but if they are present CT or more invasive procedures should be performed. The presence of bony lesions, moreover, does not correlate well with the actual extent of tumor, which is usually more important [7, 12].

II. Computed Tomography

Computerized tomography can be performed either with no additional procedure (plain CT) or associated with IV or intrathecal (IT) injection of contrast medium [2, 4, 8, 17, 22].

1. Plain CT

Plain CT is extremely valuable in demonstrating bony lesions. The visualization of intraspinal content, on the other hand, will vary according to the performance of the CT unit. Nevertheless, the spinal cord will usually be clearly visible on CT of the upper cervical level.

Further caudally the quality of demonstration of the spinal cord is not consistent. Certain tumors may be suspected, as they are naturally slightly hyperdense and show an associated enlarged medullary shadow.

Highly hypodense components, such as lipomatous infiltration, will also be clearly visible.

Cystic lesions are detectable if sufficiently large. Again, all these pathologic findings suggest the performance of more invasive or more accurate procedures, and in this way are extremely valuable in selection of patients in whom traumatic investigative procedures are indicated.

2. CT with IV Contrast Injection

Several spinal cord tumors are enhanced vividly after bolus injection of contrast medium: spinal angiomas, hemangioblastomas. Ependymomas, and especially myxopapillary ependymomas of the filum terminale and astrocytoma are also enhanced after IV contrast injection, but less intensely. We feel that CT associated with IV contrast injection will again indicate what neuroradiologic procedures should subsequently be performed. CT demonstration of highly vascularized masses calls for appropriate angiography and prevents dangerous procedures such as puncture of an enlarged spinal cord, which is sometimes advocated ("syringogram".

3. CT with IT Injection of Nonionic Water-Soluble Contrast Medium

CT with IT injection of nonionic water-soluble contrast medium (myelo-CT) appears to be the radiologic procedure of choice for the investigation of spinal cord tumors. Whether it schould be performed alone, using a minimal amount of contrast medium, or secondary to conventional myelography is an open question. As myelography gives a global view we still prefer to start with this procedure; it is extremely helpful in providing a guide to adequate subsequent myelo-CT.

As a consequence, we perform myelo-CT as an additional procedure providing information complementing that obtained by myelography. Myelo-CT offers an answer to most of the questions raised in the case of tumoral infiltration of the cord: precise tumor extent, presence of cystic or lipid components.

Even minimal changes of the spinal cord shape are precisely depicted thanks to the tomographic axial approach provided by CT.

As CT is more sensitive than conventional radiography, even a minimal amount of contrast medium is detected on myelo-CT: therefore, myelo-CT will reveal the exact extent of tumor infiltration causing a myelographic block.

Indeed, while the myelographic approach requires both lumbar and cervical contrast injection to determine the full extent of a tumor infiltration causing total arrest of contrast medium, myelo-CT can usually demonstrate both poles of the tumor, owing to its high sensitivity. As a consequence, we advocate myelography with injection by the lumbar route, followed by supplementary myelo-CT, thus avoiding a second cervical myelography.

Compared with myelography, myelo-CT allows easier differential diagnosis between intra- and extramedullary lesions. Again, the axial approach given by CT gives better visualization of the progressive enlargement of the spinal cord in the case of an intramedullary lesion. In the presence of an extramedullary lesion the progressive compression and displacement of the medullary shadow is very well visualized by myelo-CT.

Myelo-CT and delayed myelo-CT allow visualization of the intramedullary cystic components frequently associated with tumor infiltration of the spinal cord. According to HAN et al. [16], in all cases of syrinx associated with tumor studied by delayed myelo-CT there was opacification of the syrinx.

The exact mechanism for filling of a cordal cavity is not clearly understood, but transneural passage of fluid must be considered as a possible mechanism. We have observed a large syrinx associated with spinal cord tumor that was not enhanced even on delayed myelo-CT.

Hydromyelia can also be responsible for a tumor-like enlargement of the medullary shadow and be enhanced on delayed myelo-CT. Enhancement of the cavity on delayed myelo-CT does not always occur in our experience, so that it can be very difficult to detect enlargement of the spinal cord due to hydromyelia.

More experience must be gained, and at the moment differential diagnosis between hydromyelia and syringomyelic tumor on the basis of late enhancement of an intraspinal cavity can still be difficult. The presence of associated malformation of the craniovertebral region will indicate congenital hydromyelia, while an enlarged cord with an irregular outline, excentric cavities, and complete myelographic block without any associated congenital malformation will suggest a diagnosis of syringomyelia associated with tumor infiltration.

It must be stressed, and the neuroradiologist should be aware that according to Poser, 16.4% of patients in whom syringomyelia is suspected on the basis of a clinical examination, in fact have intramedullary tumors [19].

III. Myelography

Nonionic water-soluble myelography has long been considered the method of choice for the examination of spinal cord tumors. The optimum procedure at this time combines myelography with myelo-CT. However, magnetic resonance imaging (MRI), although experimental at this time, already looks like becoming the procedure of choice.

Myelographic signs of tumor infiltration include progressive spinal cord enlargement, often irregular in shape, associated with progressive obliteration of the subarachnoid opacified compartment. It must be stressed that myelography alone has its shortcomings:

widening of the cord may have a nontumor origin, as in the case of syringo- or hydromyelia. In this respect the easiest diagnostic pathway includes secondary myelo CT. On the other hand, myelography has the valuable advantage of offering a better overal view of the lesion in the absence of a total block [14, 15, 27].

Differential diagnosis of an enlarged cord must include spinal angioma: in 75% of spinal angiomas serpiginous negative filling defects are seen on myelography and are highly suggestive. Nevertheless it must be stressed that in 25% of spinal angiomas myelography may be nondiagnostic. On the other hand, enlarged, tortuous spinal cord vessels may accompagny myelographic obstruction due to tumor infiltration of the cord. If enlarged vessels are suspected on myelography, spinal angiography should be performed to rule out the presence of an angioma.

Gas myelography should also be mentioned as a possible and valuable diagnostic procedure: nevertheless it is a very painful examination. Associated tomographic cuts are necessary, accounting for a high level of irradiation. In addition, general anesthesia is required, so that this procedure is a very elaborate one exposing the patient to a great deal of stress.

IV. Spinal Angiography

This highly sophisticated procedure requires adequate equipment and well-trained radiologists. Nevertheless, selective spinal angiography is mandatory each time an angioma is suspected. The site and nature of the arterial feeders must be showed by selective angiography [9, 24].

The extent of the malformation and its relationship with the spinal cord must be clearly evaluated. In contrast to tumor infiltration, arteriovenous malformations seldom produce total obstruction. In the case of a spinal tumor, angiography may help the neurosurgeon to visualize the extent of vascularization and to indicate the normal arterial supply routes of the medulla (localization of the Adamckiewicz artery).

Some tumors, such as hemangioblastoma, are richly vascularized: in these cases angiography must be performed to confirm the diagnosis and to determine what neurosurgical procedure is required.

V. Spinal Phlebography

The use of spinal phlebography has also been advocated for presurgical evaluation of epidural venous compression associated with spinal cord tumors. This type of examination gives only indirect indications of tumor extent and is currently seldom applied if CT can be used.

VI. Magnetic Resonance Imaging

The new diagnostic modality of magnetic resonance imaging (MRI) will undoubtedly soon replace most of the very invasive and traumatic procedures used up to now to evaluate spinal cord lesions. Our initial experience with MRI using a superconducting 0.5 Tesla Gyroscan is extremely encouraging. If adequate head coils are used MRI gives excellent images of the cervical spinal cord. Images of the thoracolumbar region obtained with a total-body imager were more disappointing, as spatial resolution is inadequate for accurate visualization of the spinal cord. Nevertheless, cervicothoracic syringomyelia could be demonstrated very satisfactorily (Fig. 4).

The use of appropriate surface coils offers an adequate imaging modality for examination of the spinal canal.

MRI is so far considered noninvasive and harmless. Since it provides such perfect "anatomic" visualization of the spinal cord it will become the primary diagnostic imaging modality for spinal lesions when readily available clinically. The precise tumor location and extent are clearly seen. Two imaging modalities may be used: Inversion-recovery (IR) or spin-echo technique. The IR technique places more emphasis on T1 (longitudinal relaxation time); with this modality spinal fluid is clearly seen and the spinal shape is superbly demonstrated. Intraspinal cysts show up distinctly. With the spin-echo technique the images obtained depend more on T2 (transverse relaxation time) when long repetition times are selected (2000 à 5000 msec); spinal cord and fluid are sometimes indistinguishable, and tumorous infiltration is very well visualized as areas of high intensity owing a prolonged T2.

Although our experience is still limited, we feel that MRI will definitely replace myelography and myelo-CT for the study of spinal cord tumors.

Moreover, it must be stressed that MRI can be performed as an out-patient technique. Unlike myelography, MRI involves no risk of worsening the patient's condition.

As a consequence, we feel that MRI must be used as the first and often the only imaging modality whenever a spinal cord lesion is suspected. At this time, an early diagnosis is possible as MRI appears to be very sensitive. There is no doubt but that MRI will help us to a new and better understanding of spinal cord disease [13, 16, 18, 21, 30].

C. Intramedullary Tumors

Tumor infiltration of the spinal cord causes enlargement of the medullary shadow. Nevertheless, it should be borne in mind that in most cases swelling of the spinal cord is due to syringomyelia or hydromyelia [3, 6, 29].

Enlargement of the cord linked with tumor is usually irregular in shape, and axial cuts of the cord reveal a rather excentric location of the mass. Wormlike blood vessels may be observed on the cord's surface. Complete myelographic block and absence of congenital skeletal abnormalities are features suggestive of a tumorous etiology of medullary enlargement.

In contrast, when tumor infiltration is suspected a histological diagnosis is often impossible on the sole basis of the radiologic findings. Location, extent, and appearance together with the clinical history will be very helpful in suggesting the histological nature of any particular tumorous condition.

Specific diagnosis is only possible for lipomas that present a specific low-density appearance on CT and for hemangioblastomas with their typical appearance on CT combined with IV contrast enhancement and on angiography.

Intraspinal neoplasms account for 15% of all primary tumors of the CNS and its sheath elements [1, 26]. According to RUBINSTEIN [26] the incidence of primary intraspinal intramedullary gliomas is as follows: Ependymomas, 63.0%; astrocytomas (grades 1, 2), 24.5%; glioblastomas (astrocytomas grades 3, 4), 7.5%, oligodendrogliomas, 3%; other tumors, 2%. Intramedullary metastasis of intracerebral tumors or other primary tumors may be found: diagnosis of these may present severe radiologic problems.

Differential diagnosis of spinal cord enlargement must consider hydromyelia, syringomyelia, inflammatory lesions, demyelinization, postradiotherapy swellings at a certain moment of evolution, abscess, and arteriovenous malformation. Some of these diseases only present with a very specific clinical history, which makes for an easy diagnosis [20, 28].

I. Ependymomas

The ependymoma (Figs. 1–4) is the most frequent spinal tumor, accounting for 63% of primary intramedullary gliomas [26]. There is a slight male preponderance. These tumors usually occur between the 3rd and 6th decades of life. Ependymomas are slow-growing tumors: clinically they can be silent for a long period. Their extension into the spinal cord can be massive and involve more than ten spinal segments. Several histological varieties have been described. Radiologic signs include aspecific spinal cord enlargement leading to myelographic block at a late stage of evolution. Plain x-ray films may show changes caused by chronic raised pressure. On plain CT, ependymomas appear slightly hyperdense, and they are enhanced by IV injection of contrast medium. As ependymomas are highly vascular lesions spontaneous subarachnoid hemorrhage can occur. Myelo-CT and MRI will give the best visualization of the tumor. Cystic degeneration occurs in 46% of these tumors [1]. Delayed myelo-CT may show unpredictible, not constant enhancement in cystic parts of the tumor: these cysts are often excentrically sited. According to various authors, ependymomas originate most frequently (37%–60%) in the lumbar or sacral region. Many occuring in the filum terminale or conus are myxopapillary or papillary ependymomas.

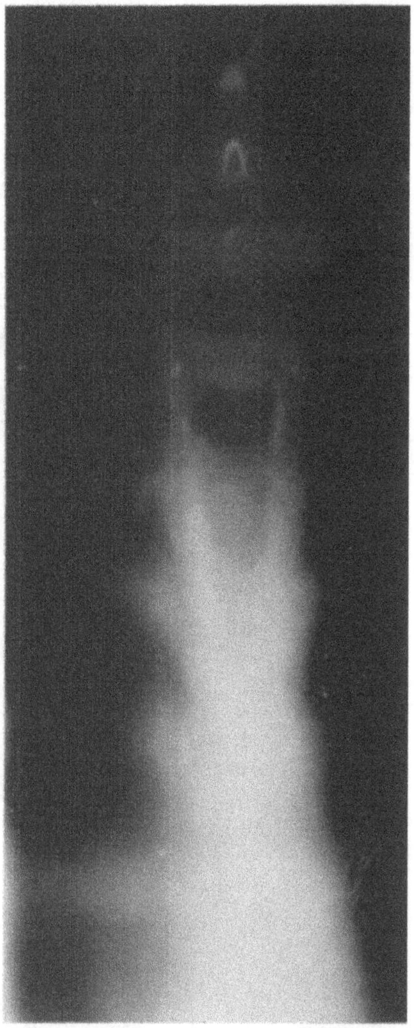

Fig. 1. Myelography of an ependymoma: frontal tomograph giving best visualization of progressive spinal cord enlargement and arrested passage of contrast medium before T4

These histological types are responsible for specific enlargement of the spinal canal lumen: they are hyperdense and are enhanced vividly in an irregular but significant way after IV contrast injection. Myxopapillary ependymomas of the filum terminale are slow growing and produce spectacular bony changes (Fig. 5).

The majority of ependymomas are benign, but extraneural metastasis has been well documented in a few cases.

II. Astrocytomas

20%–25% of intraspinal tumors are astrocytomas (Fig. 6), and 75% of these are benign [1]. There is a

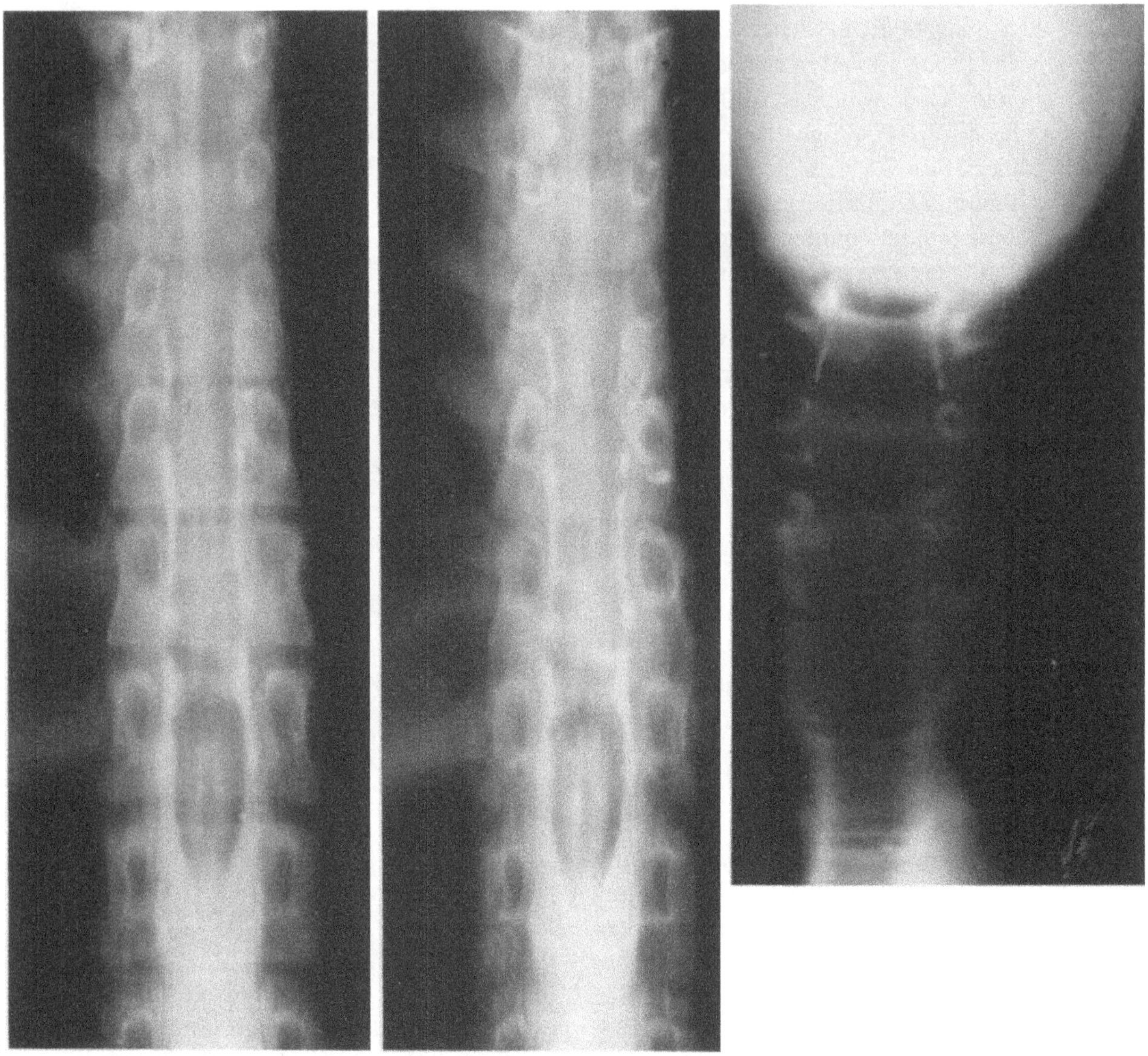

a b

Fig. 2a, b. Ependymoma infiltrating from C3 to conus medullaris. **a** Myelography with contrast injected by lumbar route revealed progressive enlargement of spinal cord and serpiginous filling defects suggestive of enlarged vessels; **b** upper cervical myelography showed upper limit of tumor infiltration in front of C3

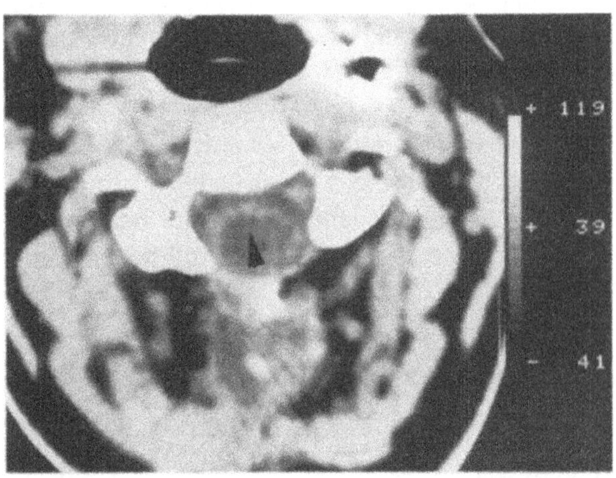

Fig. 3. Cervicothoracic ependymoma: CT following IV injection of contrast medium. Medulla is enlarged; enhancement of tumor allows better visualization of the cystic extentric component (*arrowhead*)

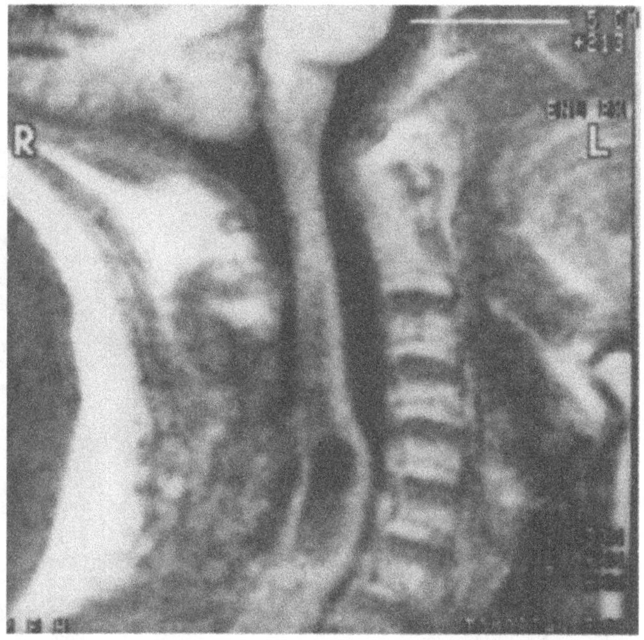

Fig. 4. Cervicothoracic ependymoma examined by MRI, revealing enlarged spinal cord in cervical area (C1 to T1). Pluricystic components within the tumorous infiltration are best visualized in this enlargement (confirmed at surgery)

slight male preponderance and they occur most often within the 3rd to 5th decades of life. The thoracic section of the cord is the most common site of these tumors, followed by its cervical section. A cystic component is observed in 38% of cases. Widening of the interpedicular distance is occasionally observed. On CT, increased density is found on plain films, and following administration of IV contrast medium astrocytomas may be enhanced (Fig. 7).

On myelography, progressive enlargement of the medullary shadow is observed without specific alterations. MRI appears to be a superior imaging modality as it is a totally atraumatic examination giving an accurate picture of the total extent of tumor infiltration. Cystic components are also well visualized on MRI.

III. Hemangioblastomas

Hemangioblastomas (Figs. 8 and 9) account for 1.6%–3.6% of all spinal tumors [26], and 20% of them are multilocular. In 60% there is an intramedullary location, and they affect the thoracic cord in 50% of cases and the cervical section in 40%. One third of hemangioblastomas are associated with Von Hippel-Lindau disease. These tumors are very frequently associated with cystic components (43%–60%).

Plain x-ray films may reveal widening of the vertebral canal. CT without IV contrast medium is usually nondiagnostic. After IV contrast injection, however, hemangioblastomas are vividly enhanced. The limits of the tumor are sharply demarcated. Myelography and myelo-CT provide less specific information: progressive enlargement of the cord is shown. Associated serpiginous filling defects may suggest the highly vascular nature of the tumorous enlargement. MRI is highly sensitive to flow phenomena and in this respect shows very specific signal alterations with spinal hemangioblastoma. Being atraumatic compared wich other imaging modalities, MRI again appears to be the method of choice for detecting spinal cord tumors. Nevertheless, angiography is still mandatory in the case of hemangioblastomas: the precise feeding vessels of the tumor must be identified to allow neurosurgical treatment. The angiographic appearance of hemangioblastomas is also very specific, allowing a definite diagnosis for this type of spinal cord tumor [20].

IV. Lipomas

Lipomas (Fig. 10) account for 1% of spinal intradural tumors. They affect both sexes equally. They can be located subpially along the spinal cord, in

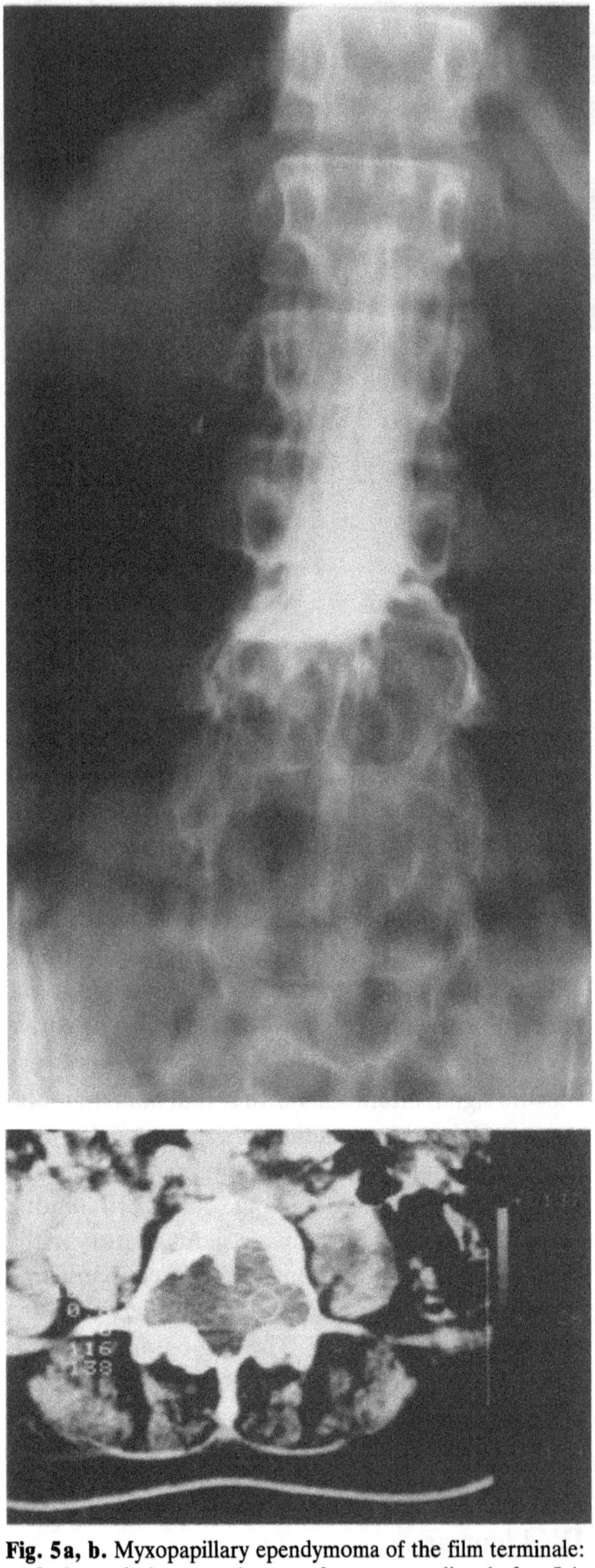

a

b

Fig. 5 a, b. Myxopapillary ependymoma of the film terminale: **a** Myelograph shows total arrest of contrast medium before L4, with typically associated erosion of L4 and L5 and of the upper sacral region. **b** CT with IV contrast enhancement shows enlargement of the canalar lumen occupied by heterogeneously hyperdense tumor with irregular uptake of contrast medium

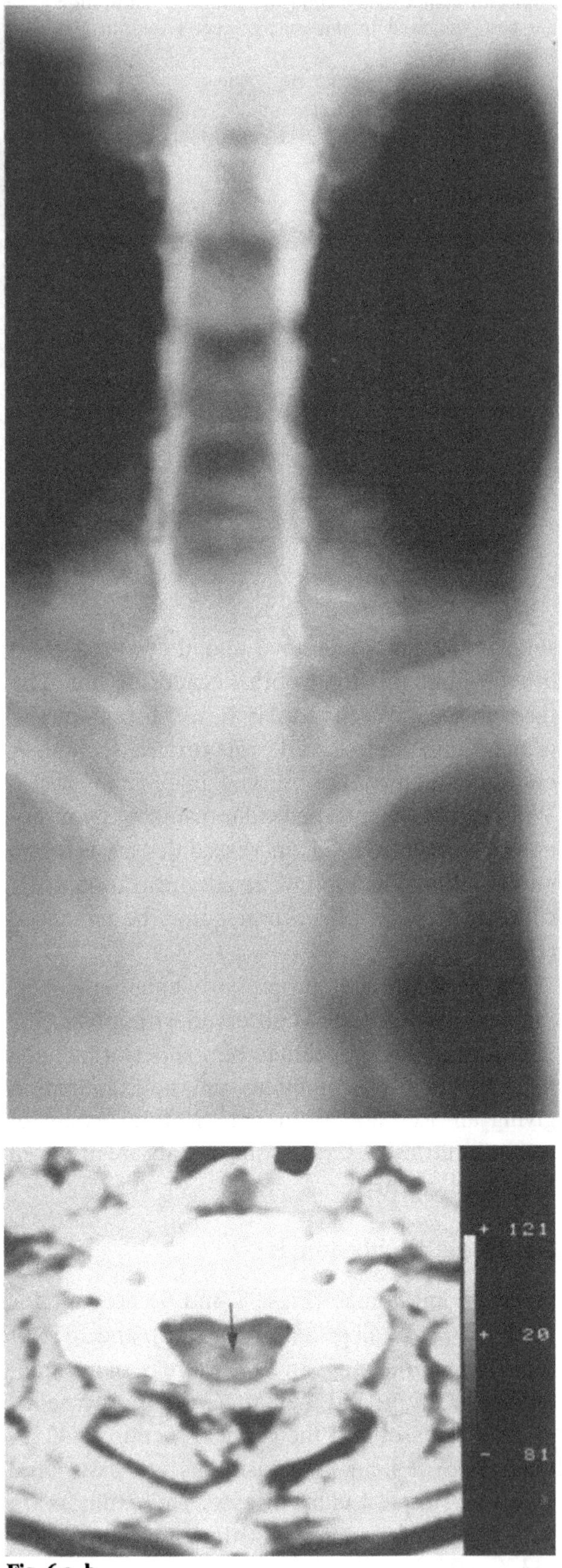

a

b

Fig. 6 a, b

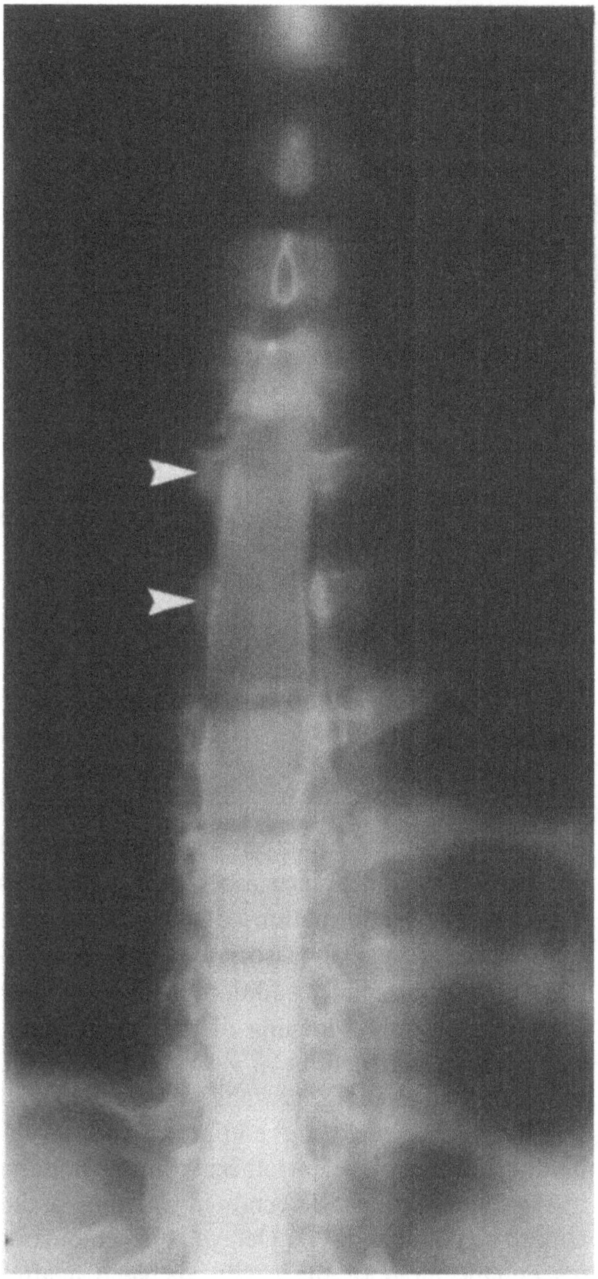

Fig. 7. Myelography in a glioma, showing progressive enlargement of the middle thoracic region of the spinal cord. Frontal tomography providing excellent delineation of extent of tumor and demonstrating associated, widening of transverse diameter of spinal capal owing to symmetrically eroded pedicles (*arrows*). No myelographic block

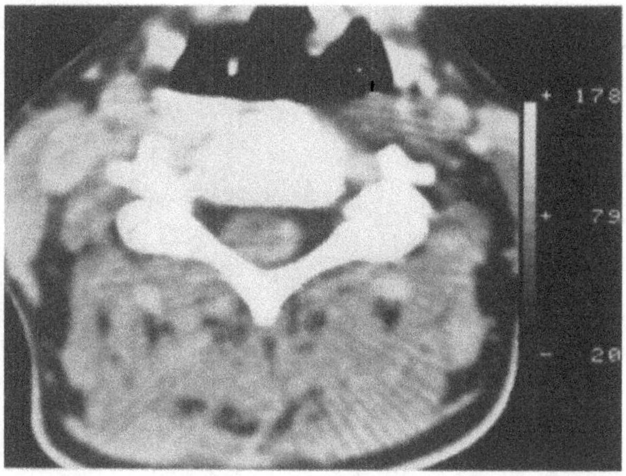

a

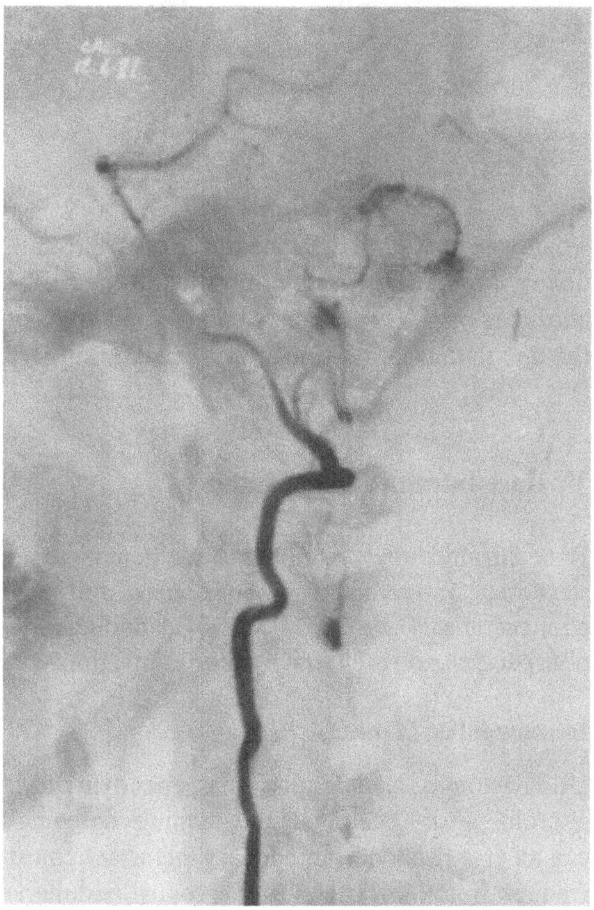

b

Fig. 8a, b. Cervical hemangioblastoma (von Hippel-Lindau disease). **a** CT with IV injection of contrast medium shows tumor with sharply demarcated margins and vividly enhanced. **b** Vertebral angiograph shows tumor vascularization of cervical and multiple posterior fossa lesions. (Courtesy of Prof. J. J. Merland, Paris)

◁ **Fig. 6a, b.** Astrocytoma. Myelography (**a**) shows enlarged spinal cord in lower cervical and upper thoracic regions; myelo-CT confirmes enlargement of the medullary shape. The cystic component (*arrow*) already seen on plain CT (**b**) does not enhance even on delayed myelo-CT

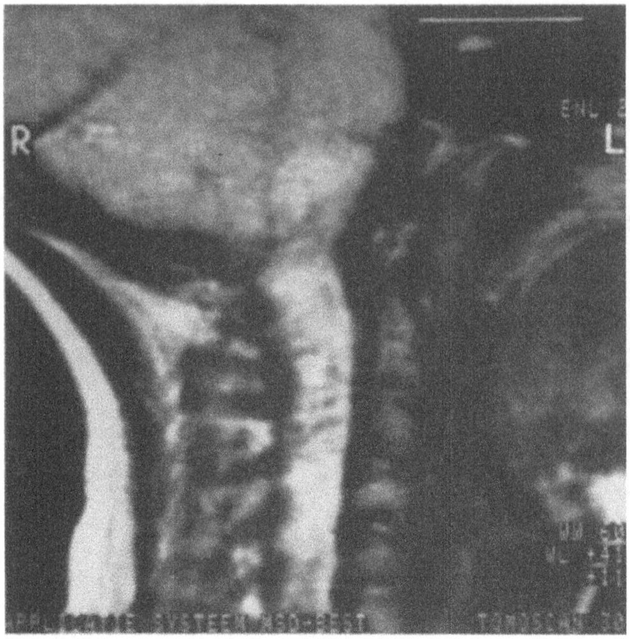

Fig. 9. Cervical hemangioblastoma demonstrated by MRI

which case they have the appearance of an intramedullary tumor. True fatty infiltration of the spinal cord may occur: in these cases no defined limits of the lipomatous infiltration are revealed on surgery (Fig. 10b).

V. Rare Intramedullary Tumors

Rare intramedullary tumors include hemangiopericytomas, intramedullary neurinomas, and ganglioneuromas (Fig. 11). Radiologic findings are nonspecific and reveal only tumor infiltration.

Intramedullar Metastasis

Glioblastomas, medulloblastomas, ependymomas, choroid plexus pailloma, and meningiosarcomas can all give rise to intramedullary metastasis, most frequently (50%) affecting the conus medullaris and cauda equina (Fig. 12).

Intramedullary metastases are often undetected unless or until an autopsy is performed. The tiny nodular intramedullary infiltrations are located mainly within the posterior part of the medulla. Radiologically they are very difficult to see, except when they produce myelographic block. Again, MRI can be expected to provide an optimal diagnostic procedure [15].

VI. Differential Diagnosis of Enlarged Spinal Cord

Hydromyelia frequently leads to an enlarged appearance of the medulla although flattening and an "atrophic" appearance aspect are sometimes encountered. Malformations of the craniovertebral region are usually associated, as is Arnold-Chiari malformation. In addition, plain x-ray films often demonstrate widening of the spinal canal, and scoliosis is present in 85% of cases. Plain CT may reveal a cystic appearance of the widened spinal cord, especially at the upper cervical level.

At the thoracic level intrathecal contrast must be injected for confident detection of widening of the cord to be possible by CT. Delayed CT demonstrates enhancement of the cavity visible 6 h after contrast injection. By 24 h later the cavity only retains contrast medium (Fig. 13). It must be stressed that hydromyelia is sometimes not enhanced on delayed myelo CT.

MRI gives ideal visualization of any craniovertebral abnormalities present and of intramedullary cavitation (Fig. 14). Owing to associated scoliosis sagittal, coronal, and axial slices may be needed to obtain complete evaluation of the lesional extension.

Surface coils are needed to examine the thoracic

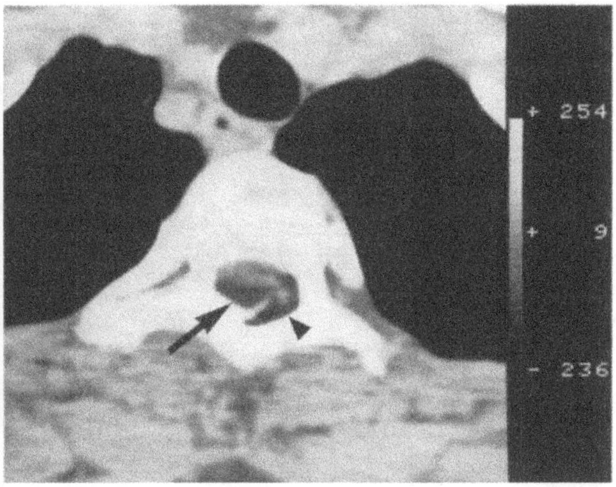

b

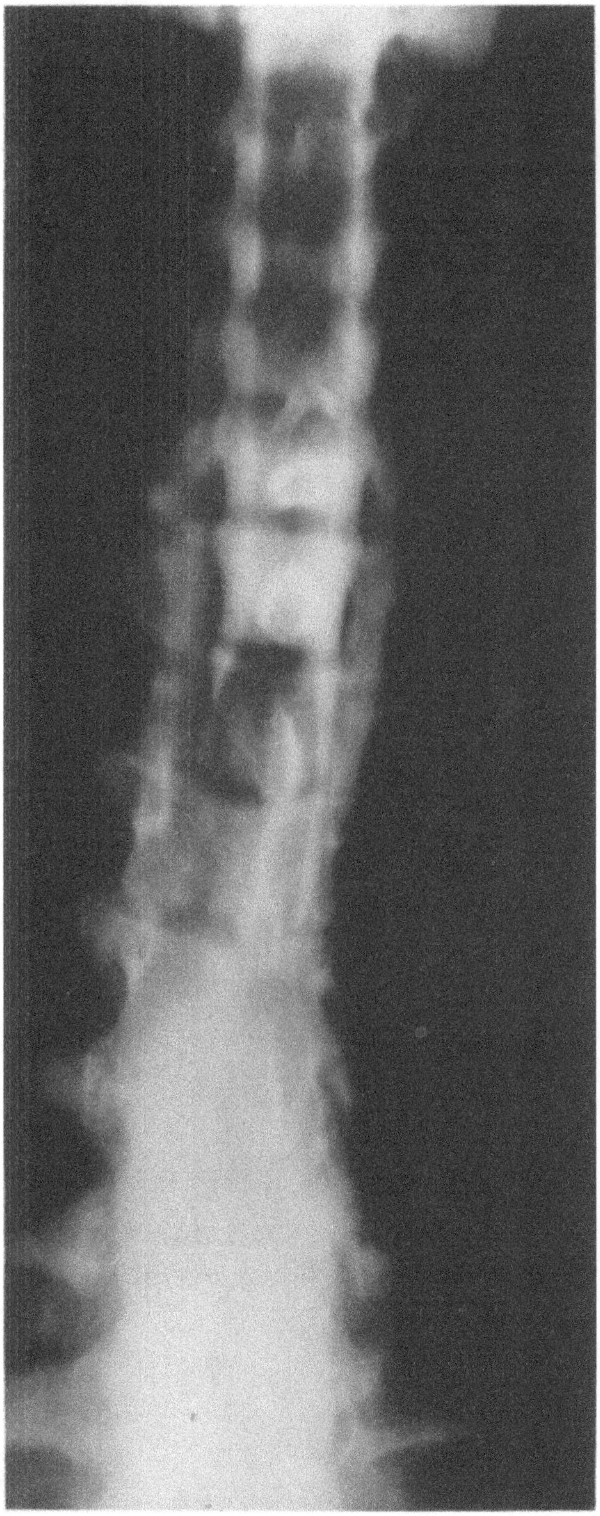

a

Fig. 10a, b. Spinal lipomeningocele: **a** Myelograph showing progressive enlargement of thoracic spinal cord; **b** only myelo-CT can show lipomatous infiltration of the medulla (*arrow*) and the associated meningocele (*arrowhead*)

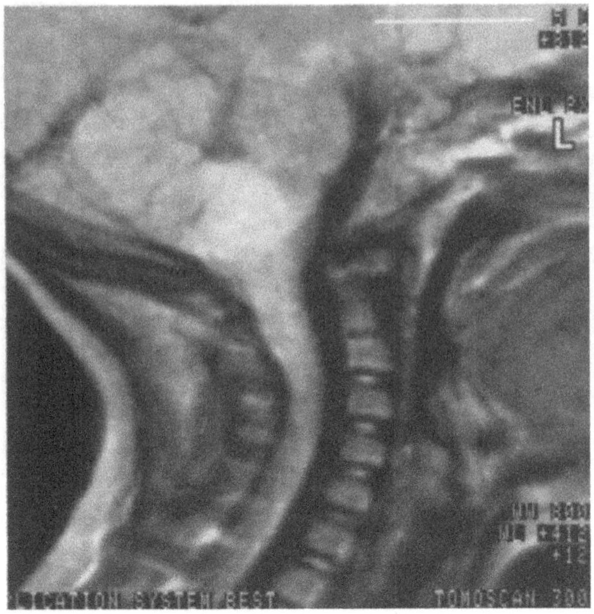

Fig. 11. Ganglioneuroma of the upper cervical region examined by MRI

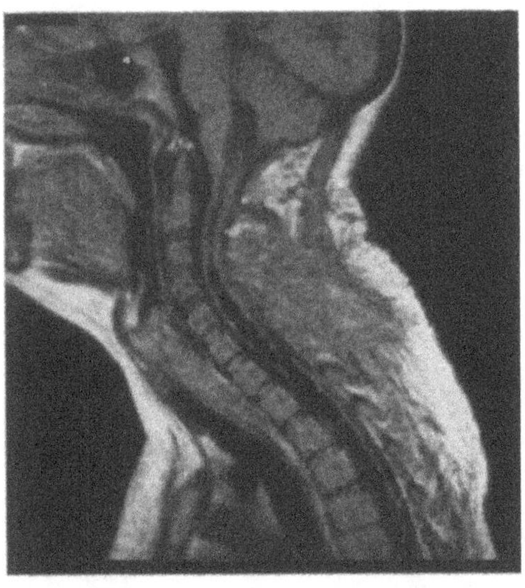

Fig. 14. MRI findings in hydromyelia: excellent visualization of the cavity by a totally atraumatic imaging modality

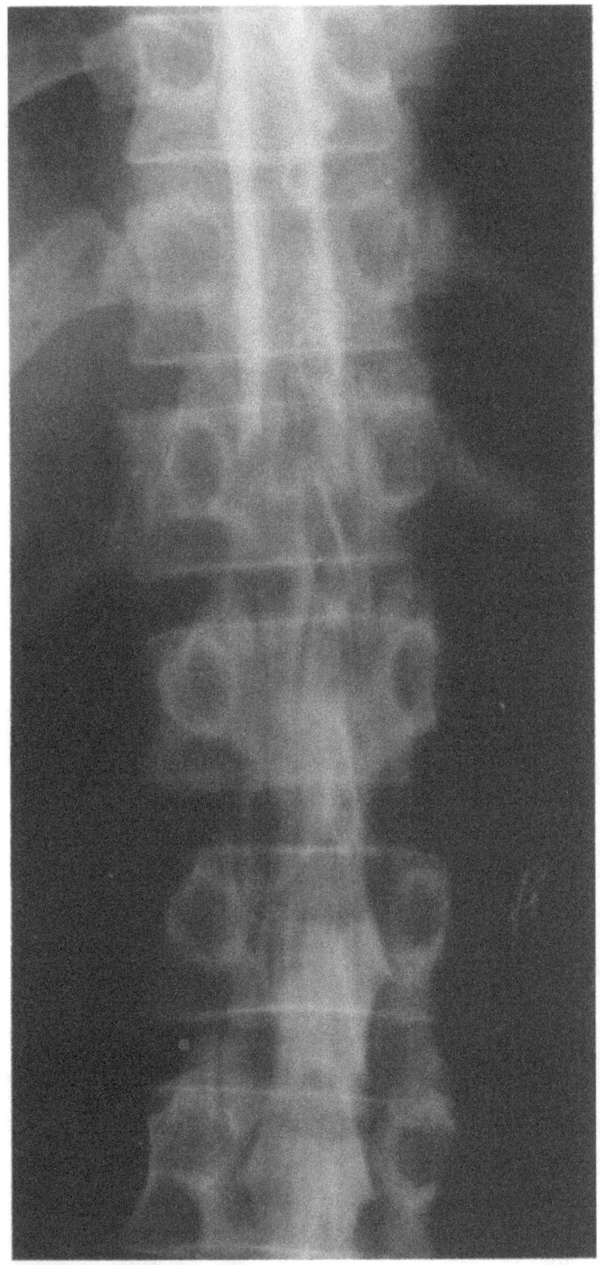

Fig. 12. Myelograph showing tumor infiltration of conus medullaris by an intramedullary metastasis of a cerebral meningosarcoma

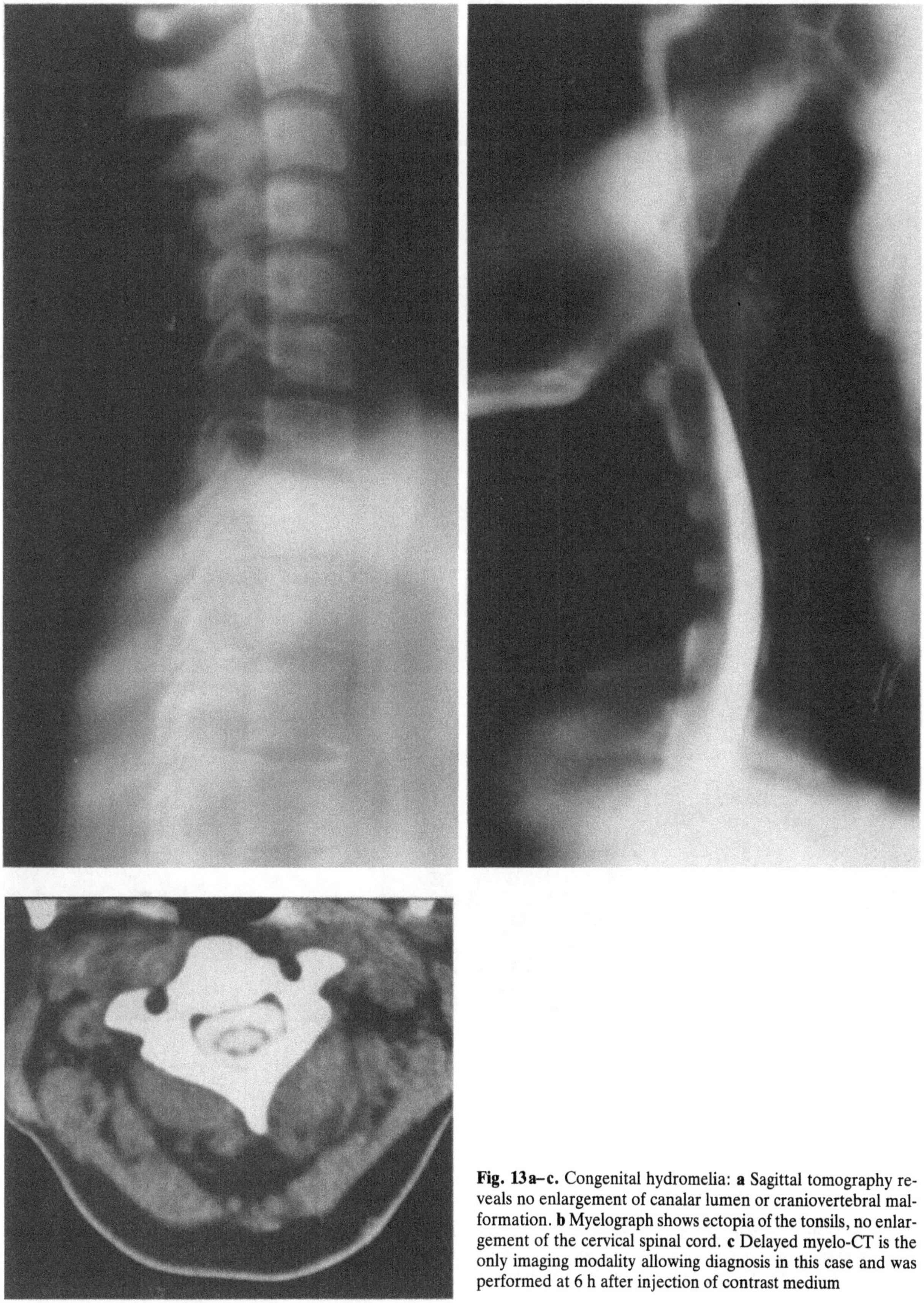

a b c

Fig. 13a–c. Congenital hydromelia: **a** Sagittal tomography reveals no enlargement of canalar lumen or craniovertebral malformation. **b** Myelograph shows ectopia of the tonsils, no enlargement of the cervical spinal cord. **c** Delayed myelo-CT is the only imaging modality allowing diagnosis in this case and was performed at 6 h after injection of contrast medium

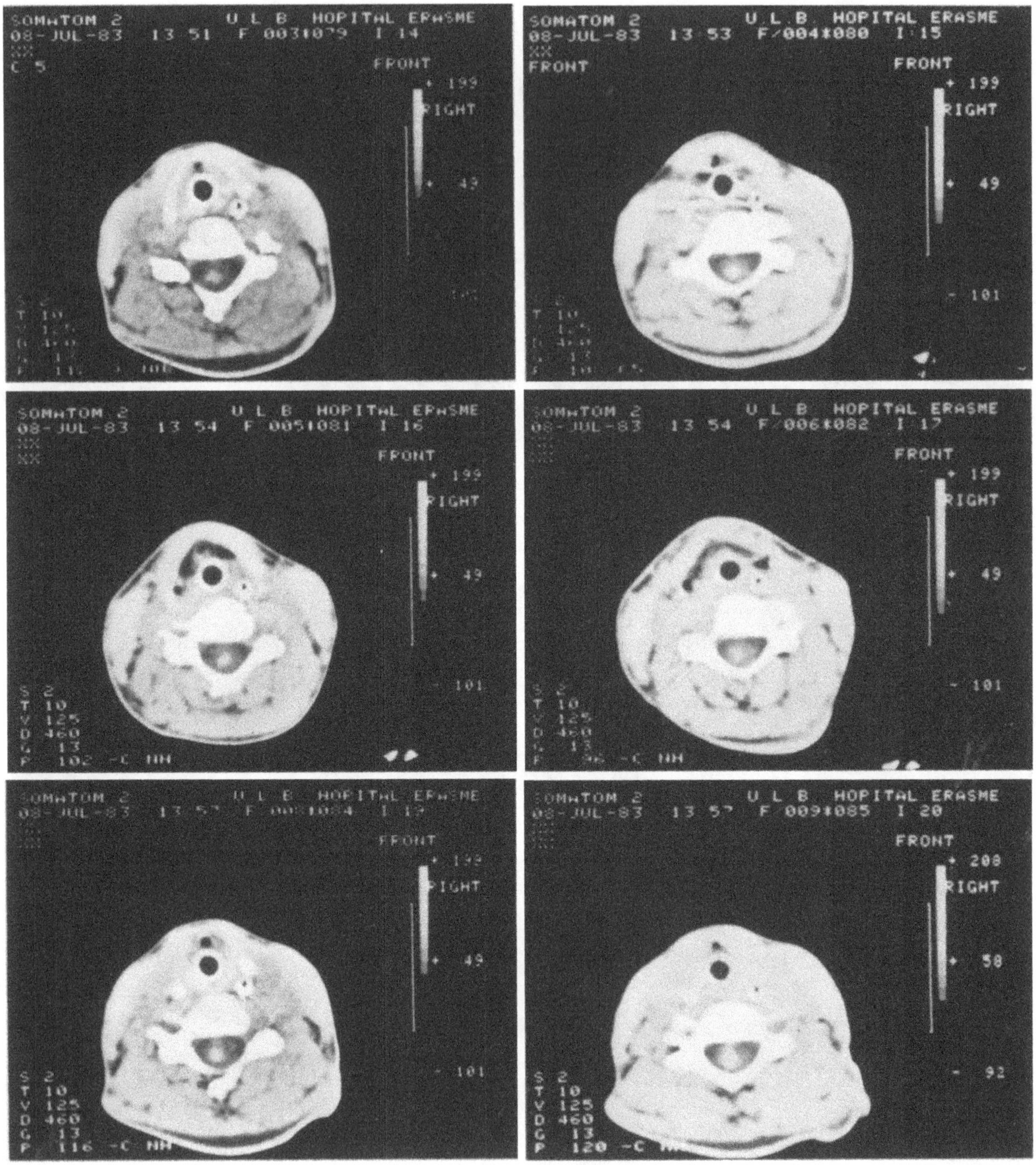

Fig. 15 a

Fig. 15. a Acute hematomyelia demonstrated on emergency plain CT examination as a spontaneously hyperdense image seen constantly and reproducibly within the spinal cord; **b** syringomyelia arising as sequela, revealed by postoperative CT examination

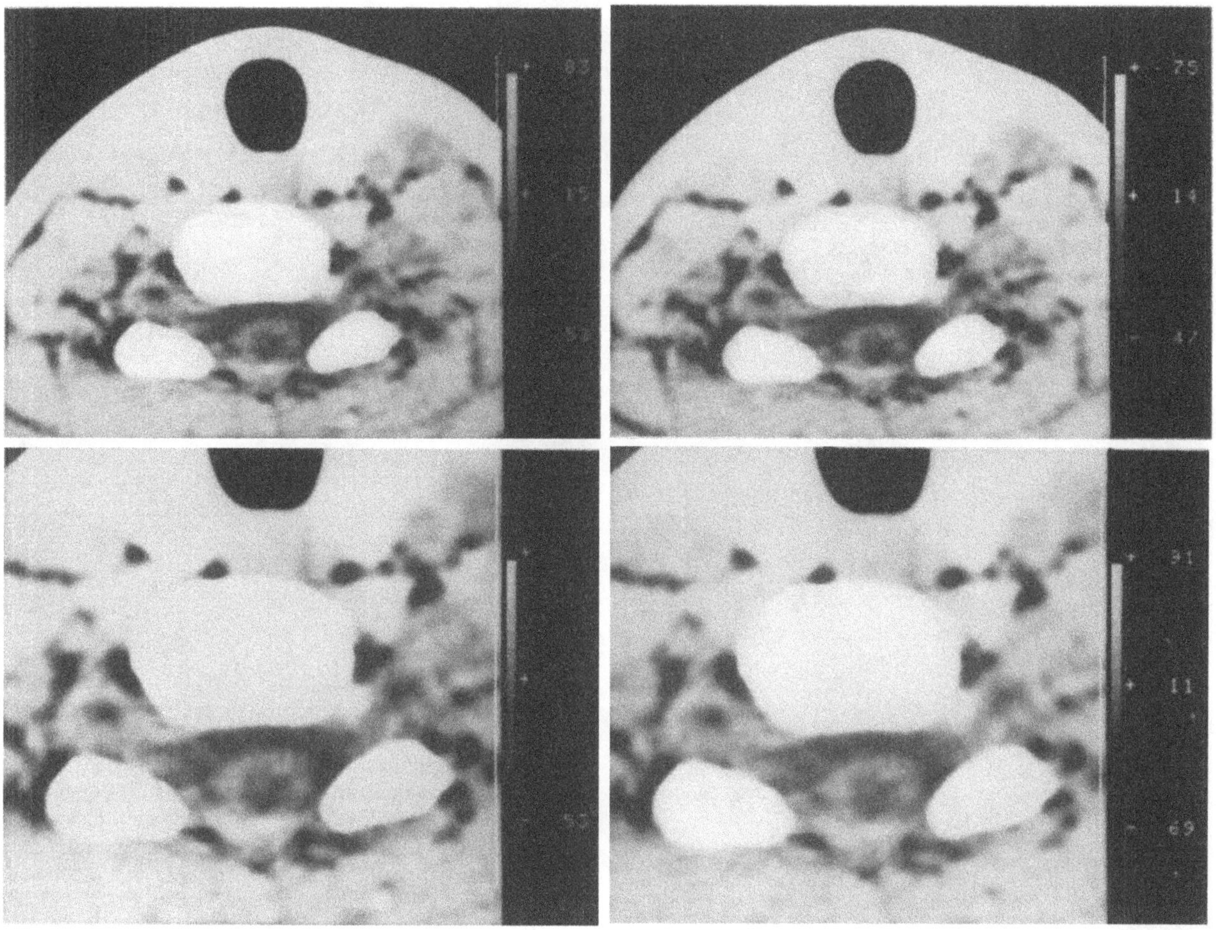

Fig. 15 b

and thoraco-lumbar levels. MRI does not provide information about the CSF circulation as myelo-CT does. In this repect, MRI and myelo-CT appear to complement each other. Syringomyelia can be observed secondary to severe spinal trauma; vertebral fractures causing narrowing of the spinal canal and medullary compression are present.

Secondary cavitation may be observed and develop several years after trauma. MRI appears to be the optimum diagnostic procedure. Syringomyelia is also found, associated with arachnoiditis. According to the clinical history, this etiology must be kept in mind. Again MRI seems to be an ideal diagnostic technique. Acute hematomyelia can be detected on CT as a spontaneously and constantly observed hyperdense intramedullary area (Fig. 15). An acute clinical onset and a typical history should lead to the performance of plain CT. Angiography must be performed in addition to search for underlying malformations.

Intramedullary abscesses have been described: they produce nonspecific enlargement of the spinal cord. The clinical history may suggest only this specific etiology. Acute transverse myelitis may cause total myelographic block, especially when underlying spinal stenosis is present (Fig. 16). Demyelinating disease and especially multiple sclerosis may be responsible for enlargement of the medulla.

Myelography and myelo-CT can demonstrate these lesions, but again MRI appears to be more sensitive and more specific.

Radiotherapy can also be followed by enlargement of the spinal cord (Fig. 17).

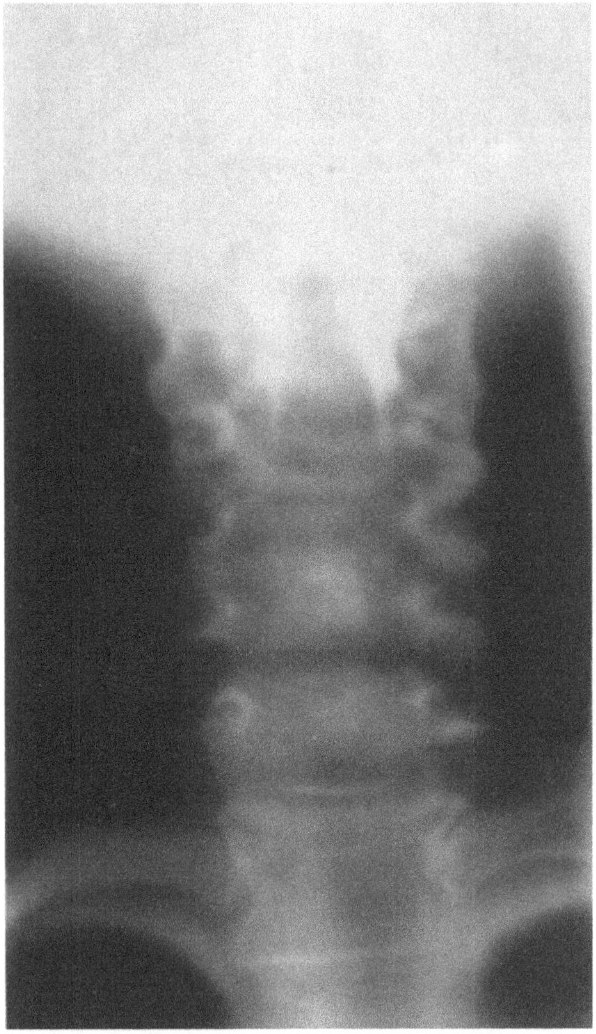

Fig. 16. Acute medullary swelling caused by inflammatory lesions of the spinal cord within a congenitally narrow spinal canal, detected on myelography and confirmed at surgery

D. Conclusion

Intramedullary tumors are rarely encountered; their evolution is usually slow.

Progressively though, they produce severe damage to the spinal cord and they cause severe disability in the patients. At this time, high hopes of being able to detect medullary tumors at an early stage seem justified. On the other hand, technical progress, including the use of Cavitron, allows the neurosurgeon to offer the patient effective treatment and complete cure of the disease.

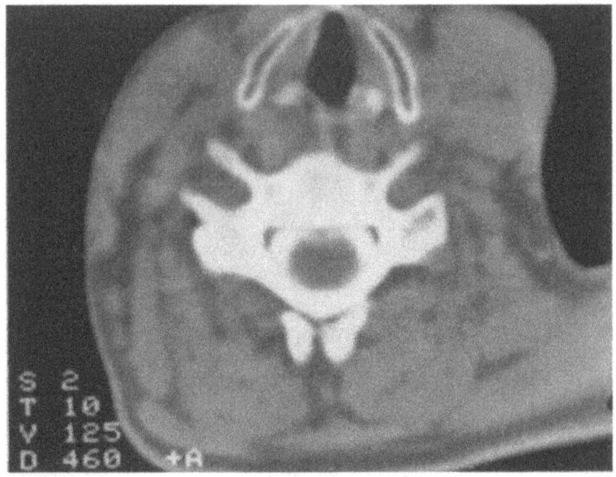

Fig. 17. Enlargement of cervical spinal cord following radiotherapy (myelo-CT)

References

1. Alter M (1975) Statistical aspects of spinal cord tumors. In: Vinken PT, Bruyn GW (eds) Handbook of clinical neurology, vol 19. American Elsevier, New York
2. Aubin ML, Jardin C, Bar D, Vignaud J (1979) Computerized tomography in 32 cases of intraspinal tumor. J Neuroradiol 6:81–92
3. Aubin ML, Vignaud J, Jardin C, et al (1981) Computed tomography in 75 clinical cases of syringomyelia. AJNR 2:199–204
4. Baleriaux D, Soeur M, Stadnik T, et al (1980) CT of the adult spine with metrizamide. In: Post MJD (ed) Radiographic avaluation of the spine: current advances with emphasis on computed tomography, chap 12. Masson, New York pp 353–365
5. Baleriaux D, Divano L, Hermanus N et al. (1983) Spine. In: Jeanmart L, Baert AL, Wackenheim A (1983) Computer tomography of neck, chest, spine and limbs, vol 5. Springer, 121–144 Berlin Heidelberg New York
6. Bonafe A, Ethier R, Melancon D, et al (1980) High-resolution computer tomography in cervical syringomyelia. J Comput Assist Tomogr 4:42–47
7. Burrows EH, Leeds NE (1981) The spine and cord. In: Neuroradiology, vol 1. Churchill Livingstone, Edinburgh, pp 481–526
8. Cacayorin ED, Kiefeer SA (1982) Applications and limitations of computed tomography of the spine. Radiol Clin North Am 20:185–06
9. Djindjian R (1968) Technique de l'artériographie de la moelle épinière par aortographie sélective. Presse Med 76:159–162
10. Dorwart RH, La Masters DL, Watanabe TJ (1983) Tumors. In: Newton TH, Potts DG (eds) Computed tomography of the spine and spinal cord, vol 7. Clavadel, San Anselmo, pp 115–147
11. Dublin AB, McGahan JP, Reid MH (1983) Value of computed tomographic metrizamide myelography in the neuroradiological evaluation of the spine. Radiology 146:79–86

12. Epstein BS (1976) The spine, 4th ed. Lea and Febiger, Philadelphia
13. Genant HK, Helms CA, Chafetz, NI, et al (1984) Spine update 1984. Radiology Research and Education Foundation, San Francisco
14. Guidetti B, Fortuna A (1975) Differential diagnosis of intramedullary and extramedullary tumours. In: Vinken PJ, Bruyn GW (eds) Tumors of the spine and spinal cord. American Elseviev. New York (Handbook of clinical neurology, bol 19)
15. Guyer PB, Westbury H, Cook PL (1968) The myelographic appearances of spinal cord metastases. Br J Radiol 41:615–619
16. Han JS, Benson JE, Yoon YS (1984) Magnetic resonance imaging in the spinal column and craniovertebral junction. Radio Clin North Am 22:805–827
17. Han JS, Kaufman B, El Yousef SJ, et al (1983) NMR imaging of the spine. AJR 141:1137–1145
18. Haughton UM, Williams Al (1983) Computed tomography of the spine. Mosby, St. Louis
19. Kendall B, Symon L (1973) Cyst punction and endomyelography in cystic tumors of the spinal cord. Br J Radiol 46:198–204
20. Kendall B, Russell J (1966) Hemangioblastomas of the spinal cord. Br J Radiol 39:817–823
21. Modic MT, Weinstein MA, Pavlicek W, et al (1983) Nuclear magnetic resonance imaging of the spine. Radiology 148:757–762
22. Newton TH, Potts GD (1983) Computed tomography of the spine and spinal cord. Clavadel, San Anselmo
23. Norman D, Mills C, Brant-Zamadzki M, et al (1983) Magnetic resonance imaging of the spinal cord and canal: potentials and limitations. AJR 141: 1147–1152
24. Pia HW, Djindjian R (1978) Spinal angiomas: advances in diagnosis and therapy. Springer, Berlin Heidelberg New York
25. Post MJD, (ed) (1980) Radiographic evaluation of the spine: current advances with emphasis on computed tomography. Masson, New York
26. Rubinstein LJ (1972) Tumors of the central nervous system. United States Armed Forces Institute of Pathology, Washington (Atlas of tumor pathology, series 2, fasc 6)
27. Shapiro R (1976) Myelography, 32nd edn. Year Book Medical Publishers, Chicago
28. Tugendhaft D, Baleriaux D, Gerard J, et al (1984) Sequential CT scanning in radiation myelopathy. J Neuro-Oncol 2:249–252
29. Wang AM, Jolesz F, Rumbaugh CL, Zamani A (1983) CT assessment of thoracic extension and of concomitant lesions in syringohydromyelia. J Comput Assist Tomogr 7:18–24
30. Yeates A, Brant-Zawadzki M, Norman D, et al (1983) Nuclear magnetic resonance imaging of syringomyelia. AJNR 4:234–237

Spinal Neurinomas

G. Sandt, M. C. Kaiser, and P. Capesius

At present, it is generally accepted that spinal neurinomas, which are benign tumors arise from the Schwann cells sheathing the axons from their exit from the pia to their terminations. Consequently they can occur on any segment of the nerve, but the present chapter is mainly concerned with the intraspinal form arising at the origin of the nerve root. These tumors have been referred to by a variety of names [8]: neurinomas, neurofibromas, schwannomas, and perineural fibroblastomas.

A. Macroscopic Appearance

Spinal neurinomas appear mainly along the distal segments of the posterior nerve roots as firm, circumscribed, rubbery white masses; they are oval or round, lobulated to some degree, and contained within a richly vascularized capsule. Unlike meningiomas, they rarely adhere to the dura, but some arachnoiditis may be found. They may also contain hemorrhagic or cystic areas. According to their localization, three different types of neurinomas are described.

Intradural/extramedullary neurinomas account for 67% of tumors arising on the nerve root. Most frequently attached to a posterior root and generally localized in the posterolateral portion of the cord, they are elongated in shape and only a few centimeters in diameter. Only 10% are found on the anterior side of the cord [5]. Intradural neurinomas are generally small (Fig. 3), but at the level of the cauda equina they can reach a considerable size.

Purely *extradural neurinomas* (16%) have been referred to as hourglass tumors, diaphragmatic sacs, and dumbbell or bottleneck tumors. An additional 16% of intradural neurinomas develop an extradural component. Tumors which cause compression of the medulla necessarily have an intraspinal component, but they can extend through a grossly enlarged foramen into the paravertebral space, eventually invading the paraspinal muscles and/or the peritoneal space. These tumors produce obvious bone changes: erosion of the pedicle, enlargement of the intervertebral foramen, posterior vertebral scalloping, and thinning of the lamina.

Intramedullary neurinomas are very rare. Ten cases of solitary intramedullary neurinomas have been reported in the literature [6]. These tumors were found in the cervical and thoracic areas of the spine, and no other clinical signs of Von Recklinghausen's disease were encountered.

B. Histology

Tripier (1878), Bard (1885), and Grall (1897) first reported that these tumors arose from the Schwann cells, and this view was confirmed by Verocay (1908) and by Francini et al. (1920). Although some authors make no distinction between neurinomas and neurofibromas of Von Recklinghausen's disease, the difference remains quite obvious from the histological point of view: Neurofibromas are composed of neurofibromatous fascicules formed by proliferating Schwann cells and perineural fibroblasts derived from several nerve roots and contained within connective tissue. Neurinomas are composed exclusively of slowly proliferating Schwann cells all derived from one nerve root. Although neurofibromas and neurinomas have much in common insofar as cellular structure is concerned, the neurosurgical problem is quite different in the two cases. It is quite obvious that neurosurgery is much more complicated in the case of neurofibromas, as nerve fibers pass through them.

C. Clinical Course

The frequency of neurinomas among spinal tumors varies around 30%. NITTNER [5] found 1129 neurinomas in a series of 2987 intradural tumors (37%). In our own series over a period of 5 years 37.5% of intradural tumors were neurinomas. The incidence of neurinomas is higher in the female sex (ratio 2:1) and they are rarely encountered beyond the age of 20. KOOS and LAUBICHLER [3] reported 17 neurinomas in a series of 205 intradural tumors in children (8.2%).

The distribution of neurinomas throughout the spine is fairly uniform with a slight predominance in the lumbar region.

I. Duration of Evolution of the Clinical History

From a clinical point of view it is quite remarkable how long a time can elapse from the appearance of the first clinical symptoms to the degree of clinical aggravation providing the motivation for complementary radiologic investigation and leading to a precise diagnosis. This may extend over some months or even over many years. On average, the diagnosis is made after 7 years for neurinomas in the cervical section [7] and after 4 years in the thoracic and lumbar sections [9]. Obviously paramedullary neurinomas are diagnosed earlier, and 50% of these tumors are treated surgically within 2 years after the onset of clinical symptoms.

II. Clinical Signs

The clinical manifestations can be difficult to evaluate; the signs presented are extremely variable as tumors can be located in any segment of the cord. Neurinomas produce slowly progressing cord compression. Symptoms are due to compression of the nerve roots and motor and/or sensitive deficits caused by compression of the pyramidal pathways. In 72% of cases radicular pain corresponding to the level of compression is the first clinical manifestation: brachialgia in 75% of cervical neurinomas, intercostal neuralgia (45% of dorsal neurinomas), radicular pain in the lower extremities in almost 100% of lumbar neurinomas [5.9]. This pain may progressively increase and nocturnal exacerbation is typically experienced. In neurinomas of the cauda equina the anamnesis generally permits differentiation of these tumors from sciatic pain due to a disk hernia. All the same, errors are possible [4], and in a series reported from the Mayo Clinic a wrong diagnosis of disk hernia was made in 29 patients (5.6% in series of 514 intraspinal tumors). We faced similar problems in 2 cases. One patient had been operated on in another hospital upon diagnosis of a lumbar disk hernia a few months before the correct diagnosis of a neurinoma was made at our institution.

The motor deficit is generally discrete and may first appear as intermittent neurogenic claudication. Physical examination is generally disappointing: stiffness of the spine and pain evoked by percussion are late signs to appear. Neurologic signs of medullar compression are discrete at this stage: paraparesis, pyramidal deficit of the lower extremities, hyperreflexia, positive Babinski's sign. Disturbances of the sensitivity should be carefully looked for. Nevertheless, the diagnosis is seldom made at this stage, and the clinical evolution progresses towards medullary involvement, which later causes total paraplegia, first spastic and then flaccid. Problems with the urinary sphincter are frequent taking the form of incontinence or urinary retention. Pain may persist or become insufferable. Sensitory disorders become more evident and an obvious sensitive level is present. Global anesthesia and flaccid paralysis can be observed at a very late stage when the medullary damage has become irreversible.

III. Examination of the Cerebrospinal Fluid

Laboratory examination of the CSF and the manometric test are essential for the differential diagnosis between intraspinal tumor and infectious or degenerative disease of the cord. Sometimes the CSF is quite characteristic, i.e., xanthochromatic with a tendency to spontaneous coagulation. Laboratory examination shows a high albumin level. In many cases the CSF is clear, but the chemistry reveals a discrepancy between the albumin level and the cellular reaction. The albumin level exceeds 0.5 g and can reach 1–2 g and sometimes even more, but there is no cellular reaction.

The results of the manometric test (Quackenstedt-Stookey) retain their full value: Normal evaluation and drop with abdominal compression, total or partial block, and a slow drop with jungular compression. Initially these disturbances may be absent. In general, paramedullary neurinomas provoke a complete block in 75% of cases and extradural neurinomas, in 66% of the cases.

D. Radiology

In the past spinal neurinomas were diagnosed mainly by myelography. Since the introduction of CT scanning the paravertebral extension of extradural neurinomas can also be precisely demonstrated. On the other hand, plain CT examination very often fails to show up neurinomas located entirely within the vertebral canal. For this reason CT scans should always be performed after intrathecal injection of contrast medium or secondary to myelography (Fig. 4).

Radiologic signs are difficult to detect on standard x-rays in the case of relatively small tumors and obvious disorders are only radiologically visible in the presence of extensive neurinomas.

I. Standard X-Rays

Radiologic signs are due to slowly progressive expansion of the vertebral canal, i.e., progressive enlargement of the dimensions of the vertebral canal while the bony structures are not significantly eroded or destroyed.

On the AP film of the spine the enlargement of the vertebral canal is seen in widening of the interpediculate distance and thinning of the pedicle. On the lateral film posterior vertebral scalloping may be seen. The extradural form extends into the intervertebral foramen and the paravertebral space, and marked widening of the foramen may be shown. Calcifications, which are more frequently seen in meningiomas, are very rare.

II. Myelography

Differentiation between the intradural/extramedullary tumors and the uncommon form of extradural neurinomas is important.

1. Intradural/Extramedullary Neurinomas

In most cases neurinomas of this type are not detected until the stage of a complete myelographic block is reached. Only rarely are they found at an early stage, when a round or oval lacunar defect is seen on myelography. Two different types of myelographic block are differentiated, according as whether they are situated in the cervicothoracic or the lumbar region. In the cervico thoracic region a cup-shaped block associated with deviation of the cord to the opposite side of the neurinoma is observed. This creates a triangular enlargement of the subarachnoid space, which may become opacified by contrast medium. The cord may be diverted laterally or anteroposteriorly. This can be visualized clearly on AP and lateral tomograms. This sign of medullary deviation is very helpful in differentiation of cup-shaped block produced by an extramedularry intradural neurinoma or meningioma from a cup-shaped block due to an intramedullary tumor: in the latter case the cord is not diverted but appears to be definitely enlarged above and beyond the myelographic block.

In cases of complete myelographic block we used to perform opacification from above and from below the tumor. This technique permits complete visualization of the extent of the tumor, and also a secondary localization may be detected or excluded. In some patients serpiginous channel-like markings are seen at the upper pole of the tumor. These markings are caused by redundant vascular structures, probably due to venous stasis (Fig. 1a).

If the neurinoma is located at the level of the cauda equina, the only sign observed is a cup-shaped block (Fig. 2), as there is no cord at this level. Sometimes a similar myelographic appearance may be mimicked by a disk hernia, but in cases of a total myelographic block due to a neurinoma the same cup-shaped appearance is seen on the different views (AP, lateral, and oblique) (Fig. 3). Neurinomas located at the upper part of the cauda equina in the region of the conus may not be

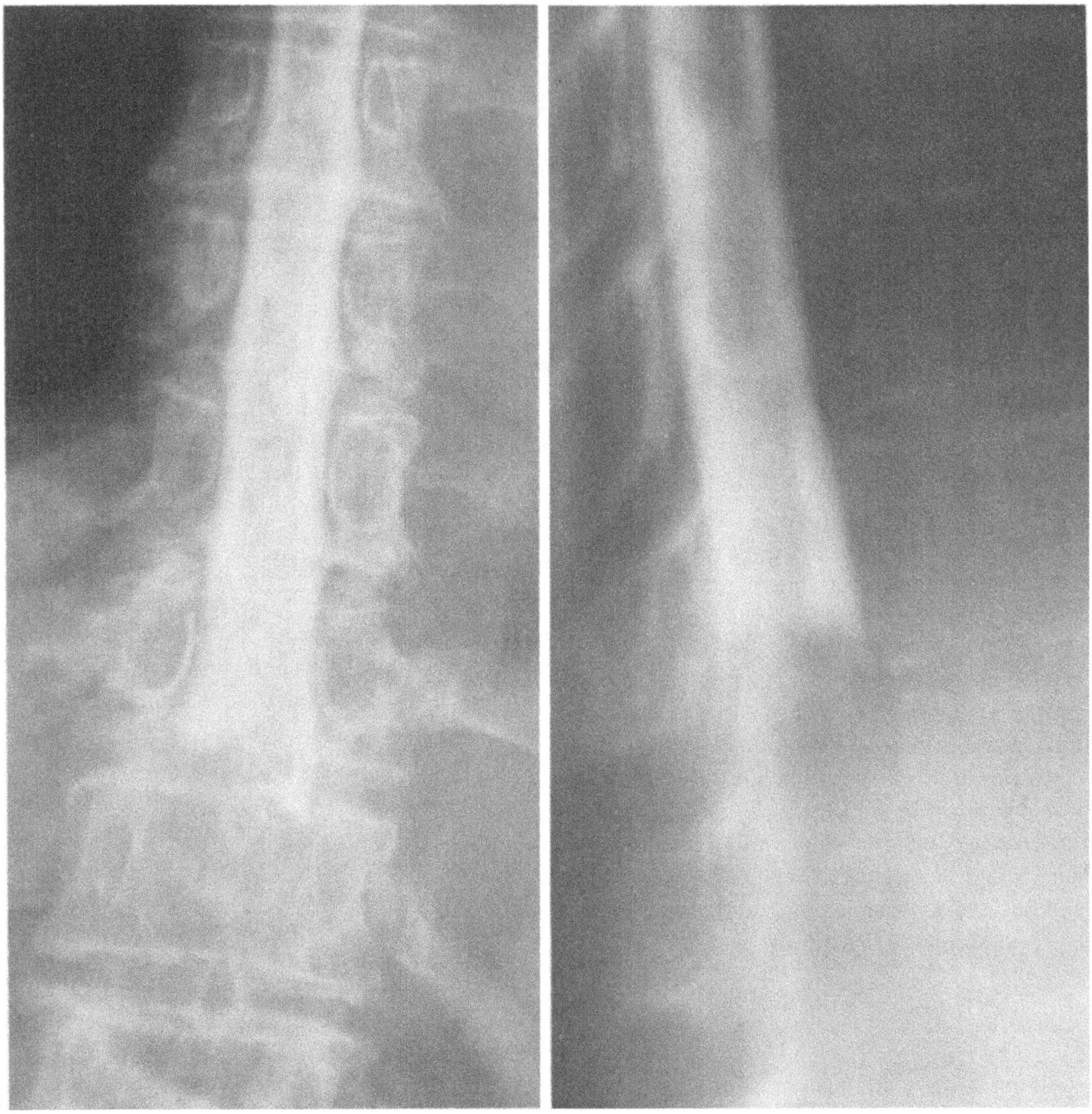

a b

Fig. 1a, b. Metrizamide myelography, AP (**a**) and lateral (**b**) views. The contrast medium was injected by the suboccipital route. Total block to progression of metrizamide outlined in the lower thoracic regiones due to extramedullary intradural neurinoma. Note redundant serpigonous veins above the upper pole of the neoplasm visualized by standard lumbar myelography, unless the table is sufficiently tilted to permit adequate opacification of this area.

2. Extradural Neurinomas

These tumors produce elongated, regular impressions of the dura. If this impression is located at the level of the center of a vertebra the diagnosis of a neoplasm is obvious. However, when this impression is localized at the height of a disk differential diagnosis from disk hernia can by very difficult. Its extension through the intervertebral foramen into the paravertebral space cannot be adequately evaluated by myelography. For this reason we routinely perform secondary CTMM in cases of complete myelographic block by a tumor. Sometimes the real nature and precise topography of the neoplasm are better demonstrated by a CT scan, but above all CT permits optimum exploration of the paravertebral extension of the neoplasm.

III. CT Scan

The diagnostic accuracy of the CT scan in intraspinal neurinomas depends to a large extent on their localization.

1. Intracanalar Neurinoma

In five cases of neurinomas detected by myelography we performed a plain CT scan at the level of the tumor several days after myelography. In none of these cases was the neurinoma detected by CT (Fig. 4). Even after a bolus injection of contrast medium no supplementary information was provided. As it is extremely difficult to obtain the exact topographic localization of a neurinoma by clinical examination alone it become quite obvious that the plain CT scan is not an appropriate technique for detection of these tumors. It is impossible to differentiate the tumor mass from the dural sac as the spinal canal may be completely filled by a homogeneous mass. Gross enlargement of the vertebral canal due to extensive neurinomas is quite clearly demonstrated by CT in the same way as by standard x-rays, but these signs do not become evident until a very late stage. For all these reasons we routinely perform secondary CTMM several hours

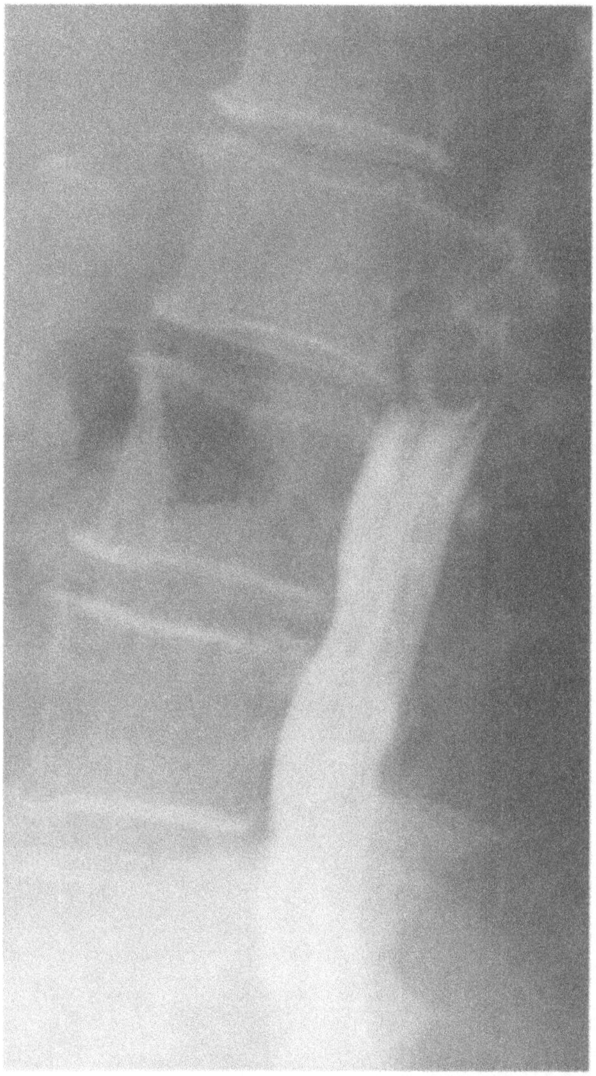

Fig. 2. Metrizamide myelography, lateral film. Contrast medium was injected by the lumbar route. Intradural mass due to a neurinoma causing cup-shaped total block to progression of the contrast medium

after myelography. Although it may sometimes be difficult to distinguish the cord surrounded by metrizamide from the neurinoma, CT has the great advantage of demonstrating the precise site and size of the tumor and its extension into the neural foramen or paravertebral space if present.

2. Extradural Neurinomas Invading the Neural Foramen

The neural foramina are very well outlined by CT scanning at the cervical level, and neurinomas can sometimes be diagnosed without intravenous and/

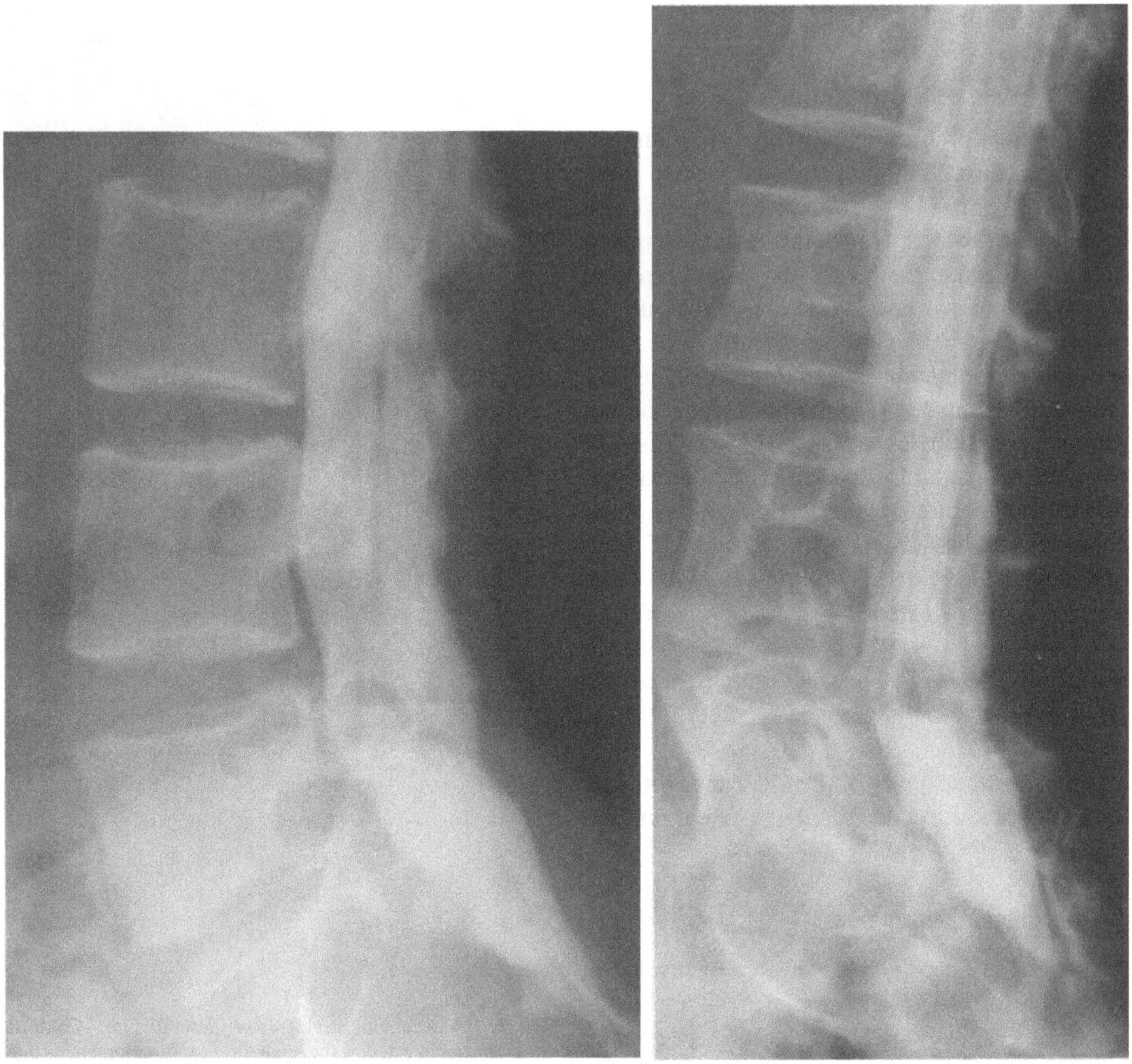

a b

Fig. 3a, b. Myelography, AP (**a**) and oblique (**b**) views. Round lacunar defect revealed at the level of L5. The lateral view shows quite marked scalloping on the posteroinferior side of the body of L5 although the tumor is relatively small. Tumor size and configuration can sometimes be shown better on oblique views. Intradural localization is clearly demonstrated

or intrathecal injection of contrast medium. At this level neurinomas are visible on plain films as round or oval masses somewhat denser than the dura and the cord. When the neurinoma is located at the upper part of the cervical spine, where the vertebral canal and the perimedullar arachnoid space are relatively large, the intraspinal extension of an extradural neurinoma can be fairly well observed on plain CT scans (Fig. 5).

3. Neurinomas Extending into the Paravertebral Space

CT is the imaging technique of choice for demonstration of the paravertebral extension of a neurinoma. In some cases these paravertebral tumor masses contain obvious calcium deposits.

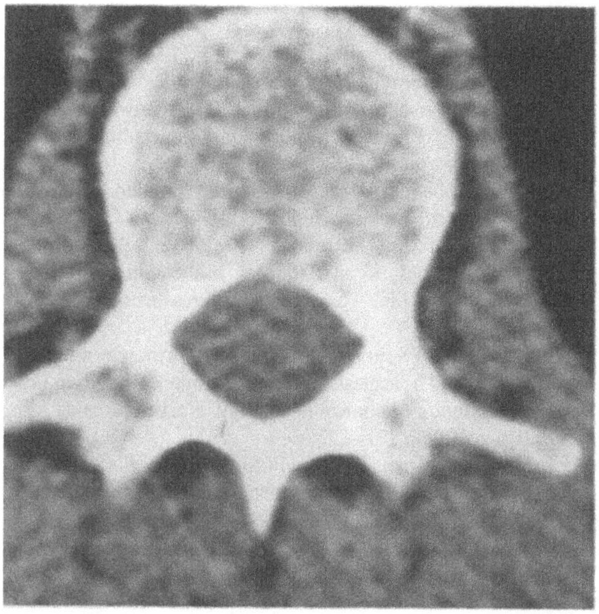

Fig. 4. Enlargement of the vertebral canal and discrete posterior scalloping outlined on the posterior vertebral wall. The canal is completely filled with a homogeneous mass, and tumor and medulla cannot be differentiated

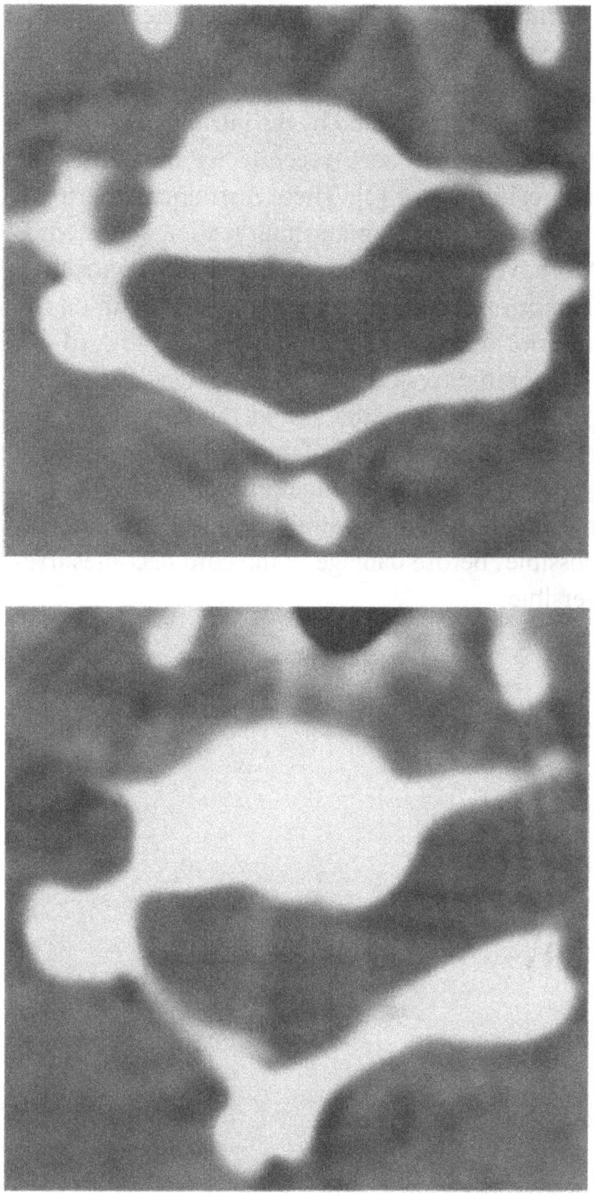

a

b

Fig. 5a, b. CT scans of the upper cervical region, showing gross enlargement of the vertebral canal (**a**) and right neural foramen (**b**). Note marked bone erosions on the right side. The diagnosis was quite obvious even without injection of contrast medium

E. Therapy

Surgery is the only way to treat these benign tumors, as pain almost always disappears after operation and permits regression or at least stabilization of the neurologic deficit. The surgical technique depends on the site of the tumor, whether it originates on an anterior or a posterior nerve root, and on its position relative to the cord and its intra- and extraspinal extension. The surgical approach is either by laminectomy or by hemilaminectomy. Once the dura has been opened the tumor is released from the nerve roots and arachnoidal adherences between the tumor capsule and the cord. The intervention should be performed with microscope monitoring. If the tumor is too large to permit easy dissection, the capsule is opened and a part of the tumor is first evacuated. After complete liberation of the tumor capsule the nerve root is dissected at its origin and the tumor is totally resected. Surgical treatment of those tumors has been greatly facilitated by the introduction of laser beams [1] and more recently by the ultrasonic surgical aspirator [2]. These instruments permit a less invasive and tramatic intervention on the cord. Moreover, hemorrhage is very easily controlled. Tumor resection is obviously more difficult on the anterior than on the posterior side of the cord.

Operative results and long-term prognosis depend largely upon the site of the tumor, but the preoperative condition of the cord is of paramount importance for the postoperative outcome. For this reason the diagnosis must be made as early as possible, before damage to the cord becomes irreversible.

References

1. Edwards MSB, Boggan JB, Fuller TS (1983 The laser in neurological surgery. J Neurosurg 59:555–556
2. Flamm ES, Ransohoff J, Wuchinich D, Broadwin A (1978) Preliminary experience with ultrasonic aspiration in neurosurgery. Neurosurgery 2:240–245
3. Koos W, Laubichler W (1967) Über die spinalen Geschwülste bei Kindern, 2. Nervenheilk. 24:247–263
4. Koyama T, Ishikawa J, Kondo A (1978) Zwei Neurinome der Cauda equina bei einem Patienten mit einem vermuteten Bandscheibenvorfall. Fallbericht. Neurochirurgia 21:172–178
5. Nittner K (1976) Spinal meningiomas, neurinomas and neurofibromas and hourglass tumors. In: Vinken PJ, Bruyn GW (eds) Handbook of clinical neurology. North-Holland, Amsterdam vol 20 pp 177–322
6. Pardatscher K, Iraci G, Cappellotto P, Rigobello L, Pellone M, Fiore D (1979) Multiple intramedullary neurinomas of the spinal cord. Case report. J Neurosurg 50:817–822
7. Piera JB, Durand J, Pannier S, Guiot G, Grossiord H (1975) Dix cas de neurinomes géants lombo-sacrés. Ann Med Interne 5:315–330
8. Russel D, Rubinstein L (1977 Pathology of tumors of the Nervous system 4th edn. Williams and Wilkins, Baltimore, p 448
9. Salah S, Horcajada J, Peaneczky A (1975) Spinal neurinomas. A comprehensive clinical and statistical study on 47 cases. Neurochirurgia 18: 77–84

Spinal Tumors in the Child

D. C. HARWOOD-NASH

The radiology of neoplasms of the spine and cord in children has evolved rapidly from a combination of standard roentgenographs, complex tomography, oily contrast medium myelography and optional air myelography [1] to standard roentgenographs, water-soluble contrast medium myelography and CT, and water-soluble contrast CT myelography alone [2].

Experience with such lesions and the modern imaging techniques, especially CT, is now also available in adults [3, 4].

A. Standard Roentgenographs

Standard spinal roentgenographs are still the preliminary examination of choice, although digital radiography may soon replace them. The latter is now often performed with the CT machine itself (Fig. 1).

Significant spinal changes are often present in both bony and neural neoplasms with significant clinical findings, but an important proportion may have disproportionate bony/neural changes and clinical alterations and vice versa (Fig. 2). In a study of intraspinal lesions in children, 30% had symptoms for less than 3 months before the definitive diagnosis is made, 50% between 3 months and 1 year, 20% for longer than 1 year. Of these children with symptoms only 50% had associated roentgenographic spinal abnormalities of any sort [1], but vertebral tumors are accompanied by roentgenographic abnormalities in 100% of cases.

Children with astrocytomas (20%) and ependymomas (67%) had *normal* spinal roentgenographs. Significant associated findings were straightening of the lumbar lordosis; scoliosis; painless torticollis; and a paraspinal mass lesion; these depended on the site and character of the underlying neoplasm.

B. Computed Tomography

Standard CT, axial CT and CT with images reconstructed in the sagittal or coronal plane or true coronal images [6] are now the techniques of choice in vertebral neoplasms. CT detects the bony abnormality and also any soft tissue component in the paraspinal space and displacement of the dural sac with intraspinal extension. There is no place for complex tomography except on the rare occasions when sagittal tomography may help. An aggressive approach is recommended in the investigation of such neoplasms, including injection of a small quantity (1–4 cm^3 isotonic) of water-soluble contrast agent into the subarachnoid space prior to CT. This means that the entire geography and character of the lesion and any significant compromise of the subarachnoid space (cord or roots) is detected at the *initial* examination. Such compromise may be considerable even in the presence of few clinical abnormalities or none at all. Intravenous contrast enhancement CT for vertebral and paravertebral lesions is also recommended after standard CT has been performed, for better determination of the bony and soft tissue changes.

Inflammatory changes often simulate neoplasia, such as Ewing's sarcoma, and vice versa. Undifferentiated sarcomas of vertebrae produce extensive and often bizarre changes (Fig. 3). Osteoma produces a dense sclerotic reaction with minimal enlargement to the affected bone; an osteoblastoma expands bone moderately and is sclerotic, often containing a heterogeneous center; an aneurysmal bone cyst (Fig. 4), however, expands bone to a pronounced degree, often producing a large eggshell-rimmed mass with a lucent center, which may significantly compromise the spinal canal. Histiocytosis X, which may or may not be a neoplasm, probably produces the most significant bony de-

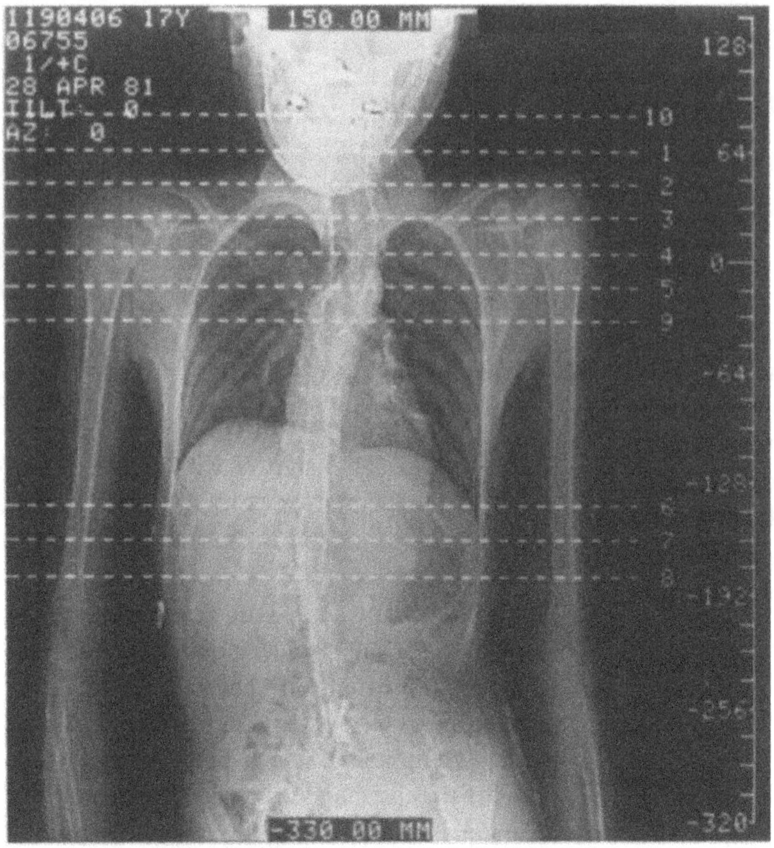

Fig. 1. Digital radiography: Digital scout view in a patient with scoliosis as a preliminary examination to CT and for prospective or retrospective slice level identification, e.g., for slice 5, as shown

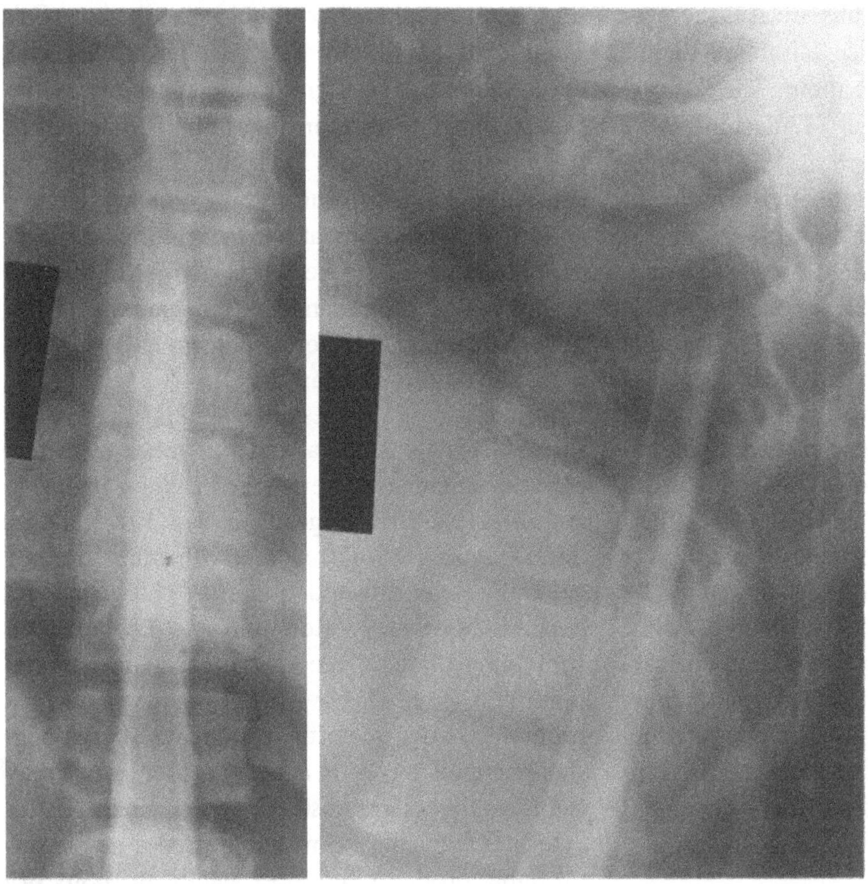

Fig. 2

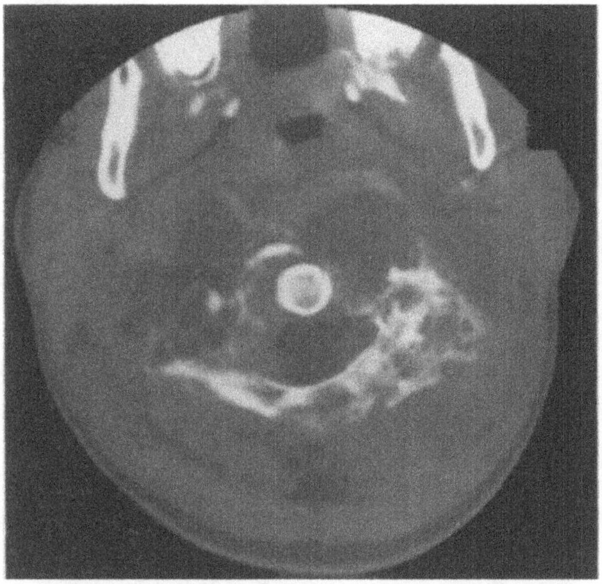

Fig. 3. Bizarre vertebral neoplasms: The destruction, expansion and surrounding soft tissue mass are clearly visualized by CT in an undifferentiated sarcoma of C2. The odontoid is intact but the dural tube (*arrow*) is distorted

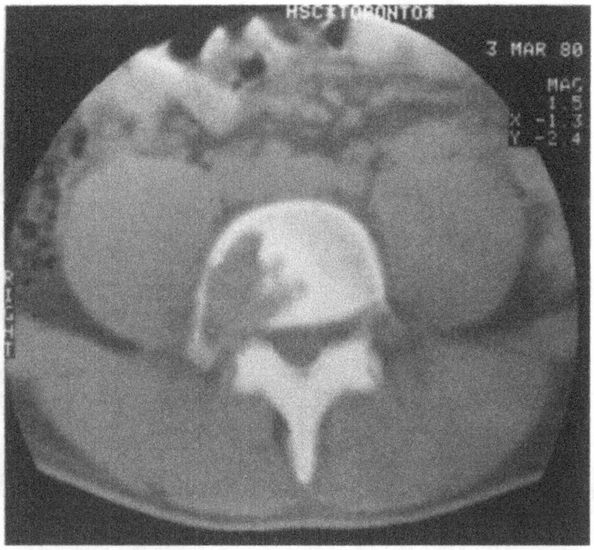

Fig. 4. Expanding benign lesion: A large aneurysmal bone cyst of L4 involving and expanding the right side of the vertebral body with the cortex still intact. The dural tube can be seen and is not compromised

◁ **Fig. 2.** Standard water-soluble contrast myelography giving a clear definition of lower thoracic and lumbar cord with a total extradural block at the midthoracic level due to leukemia. Other than a slight scoliosis no bony change demonstrated

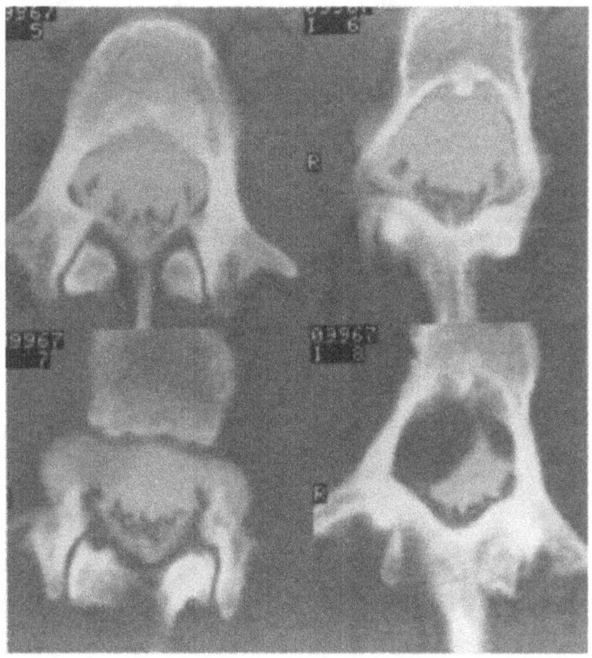

Fig. 5. Complex vertebral anomalies. A combination of CT and metrizamide clearly demonstrates the disordered cauda equina, which has a markedly widened dural sac with lateral arachnoid herniations in neurofibromatosis with associated vertebral dysplasia. Note in image 8 a large and a small associated arachnoid cyst within the canal

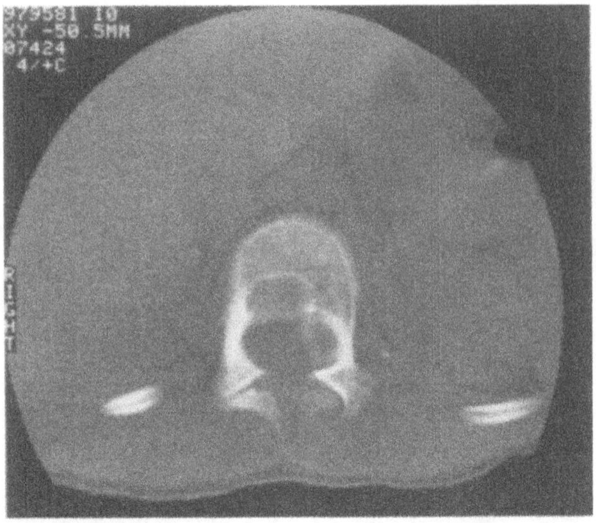

a

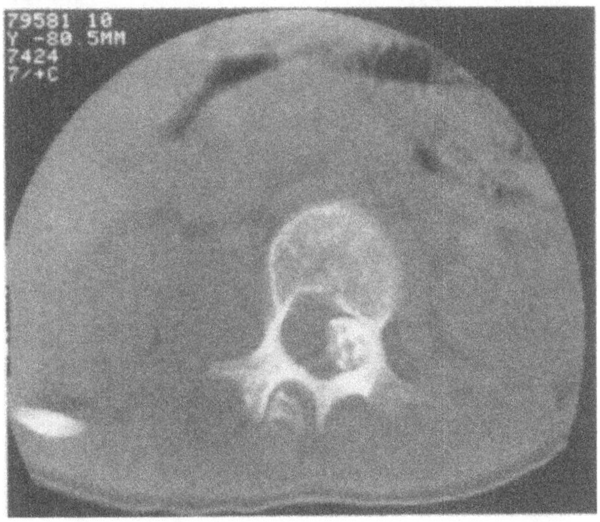

b

Fig. 6a, b. A benign chronic space-occupying mass in the extradural compartment on the right and a neurofibroma, markedly displacing the lumbar cord to the left surrounded by metrizamide (**a**) eroding its way into the vertebral body and extending to the level of the conus and cauda, again with displacement (**b**). The neurologic changes in this 10-year-old child were surprisingly slight

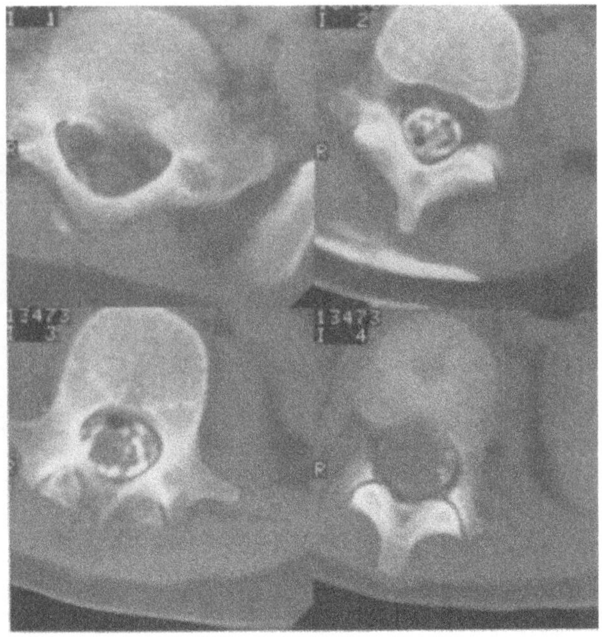

Fig. 7. Intramedullary mass lesion: An oligodendroglioma of the conus shown with CT sections from 1 to 4, passing cranial. Normal filum and cauda equina are seen image 2 with a bubble of air, an irregular conus tip in image 3 surrounded by nerve roots, and in 4 a markedly expanded irregular cord. Standard myelography showed a complete block lower than image 4; CT with contrast shows the full character of the lesion

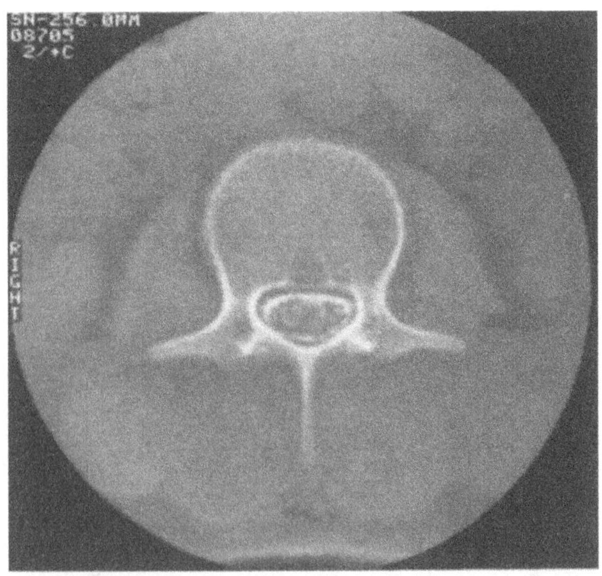

Fig. 8. Subtle cauda equina lesions: An ependymoma of the filum terminale nestling within the cauda equina and best demonstrated by CT

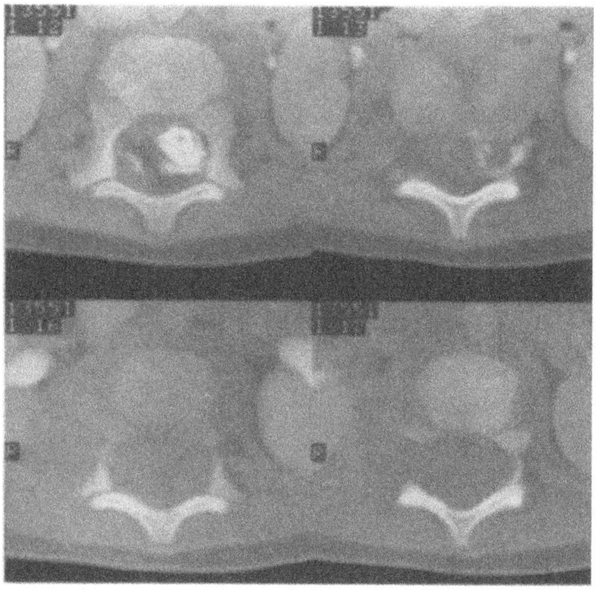

Fig. 9. Bizarre intraspinal sarcoma: CT metrizamide myelography from above shows marked displacement of the tip of the conus and cauda equina to the left (some leakage of contrast has occurred), and lower down, total obliteration of the dural sac and cauda equina to a thin rim on the left side. This child also had remarkably few distal clinical signs

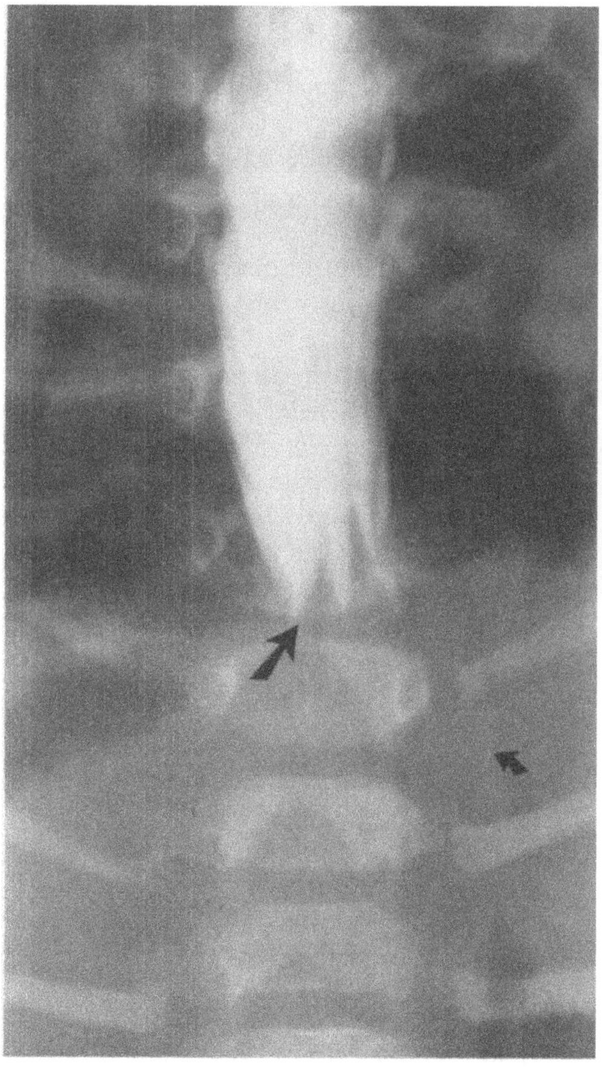

a

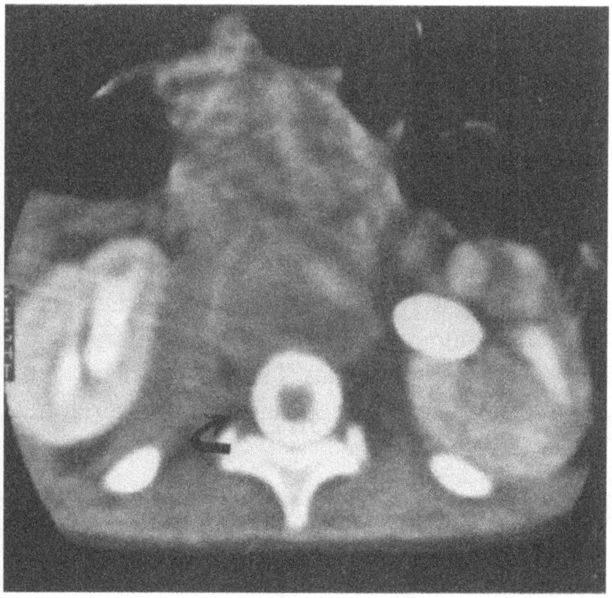

b

Fig. 10a, b. CT metrizamide myelography and paraspinal masses: **a** Standard metrizamide myelography revealing a total block in a patient with neuroblastoma with a soft tissue mass on the right side (*small arrow*) and the block predominantly on the left side in the extradural space (*large arrow*); **b** another patient, an infant with a normal myelogram and displacement of the right kidney due to neuroblastoma, demonstrating subtle intrusion (*arrow*) of the neuroblastoma to the dural sac without displacement

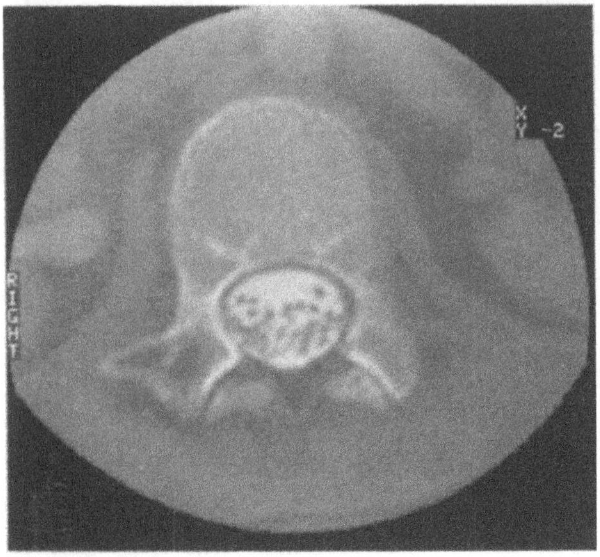

Fig. 11. Subtle intra-arachnoid lesions with disorganisation of the cauda equina and multiple nodules best seen by CT of disseminated intra-arachnoid leukemic deposits

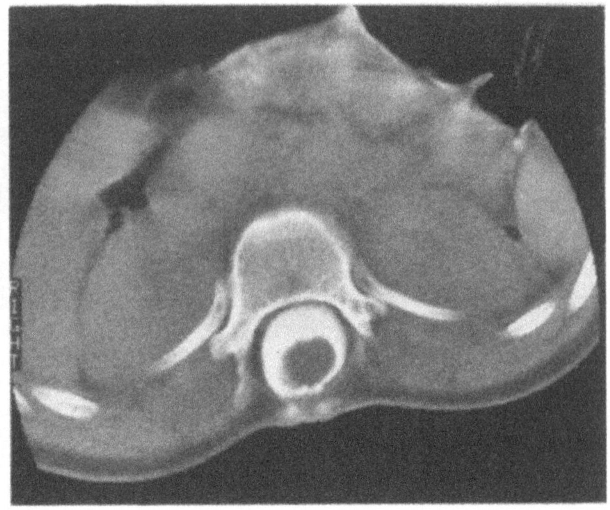

Fig. 12. A large intramedullary dermoid found in the lower thoracic spine on CT metrizamide myelography demonstrating an irregular expanded cord, a dysraphic spine, and a posterior defect with a dermoid track

struction, and its soft tissue component involves both the paraspinal and the intraspinal compartments.

Neurofibromatosis (Fig. 5) involves the vertebral bodies as intrinsic dysplasia, more often than not with dural dysplasia and a very wide dural sac with intraspinal canal enlargement. Arachnoid cysts are common within the dural dysplasia, and intracanalicular neuromas (Fig. 6) may enlarge the canal and cause scalloped defects of the vertebral body itself.

C. Water-Soluble Contrast Myelography

Water-soluble contrast agents are now exclusively used in myelography to detect intraspinal mass lesions (Fig. 2). The advantages of being absorbed, being water-soluble, having the ability to surround even large mass lesions, and being applicable to CT are paramount. The technique in children is now well established [2] and is both safe and sensitive.

D. CT Myelography

There is still no place for simple CT alone in the investigation of intraspinal canal neoplasms. The normal cord and abnormal tissue are poorly visualized below C3. It is suggested therefore that CSF contrast enhancement be used as a standard procedure.

It is best performed after a formal myelogram, although at this time CT may not define small structures and changes easily, owing to an inordinate amount of iodine in the CSF. This can be avoided in part by delaying the CT until 2–3 h after the myelogram (a secondary CT contrast myelogram), but this can involve significant logistic problems, particularly in children. An alternative is to the place a small amount of isotonic contrast agent in the CSF initially and perform a CT immediately without a standard myelogram (primary CT contrast myelogram). This latter technique is only advised after considerable experience with standard myelography and secondary CT contrast myelography, and only if the clinical and/or standard roentgenographic abnormalities are localized to a well-defined site and level in the spinal column/cord.

Mass lesions of any type, neoplastic or otherwise, are not common in children. However, of them all, developmental mass lesions (dermoid, teratoma, lipoma, neuroenteric cyst, hydromyelia) constitute 38%; primary neural neoplasms (Figs. 7 and 8) (astrocytoma, ependymoma, neurofibroma, neuroblastoma, etc.), 30%; extradural neoplasms (Fig. 9) or extension of vertebral or paravertebral neoplasms, 8%; and a miscellaneous group of disk protrusions, abscesses, etc., 14% [1].

Of spinal cord neoplasms per se, developmental (24%) and primary neural tumors (47%) were the main types in a large combined series of 364 children [1]. Astrocytomas (15%) and intraspinal extension of neuroblastomas (12%) (Fig. 10) were most common. Astrocytomas, teratomas, and hydromyelia are three lesions that can involve extensive sections or indeed the entire spinal cord, and remarkably enough, some patients affected by these present with only minimal clinical signs.

The advantage of CT contrast myelography is the full demonstration of vertebral changes, of each gross or subtle mass lesion (Fig. 11), irregular surface, any cystic component, and calcification, and a precise localization to the extradural or intradural compartment. Intramedullary lesions in children occur in 22% (astrocytomas, dermoids), intradural and extramedullary in 44% (metastases, ependymomas, dermoids), and extradural in 34% (neuroblastomas and neoplastic extension).

Furthermore, water-soluble contrast more frequently permeates even the smallest or thinnest interstices around an intradural mass lesion (Fig. 12), often giving good definition of its full extent, while standard myelography shows a complete block. Both lumbar and cervical punctures can occasionally be used in this procedure to outline the full extent of the lesion.

Intravenous contrast CT may occasionally reveal enhancement of a mass lesion, such as a teratoma or a rare malignant glioma. Arteriovenous malformations can have a very large enhancing varix with a venous type that might be mistaken for a neoplasm. Usually CSF contrast myelography identifies the abnormal smaller vessels, and subsequent angiography is essential.

E. Summary

The neuroradiological protocol followed in the case of neoplasms of the spine and cord in children must be aggressive and comprehensive.

Initial clinical and standard roentgenographic localization with CT after or primarily with water-soluble positive contrast in the CSF is the technique of choice. Intravenous contrast adds very little. In this way the complete topography and character of the lesion, possibly in one or more of the paraspinal, vertebral, extradural, intradural, or intramedullary compartments, can be quickly and accurately ascertained.

References

1. Harwood-Nash DC, Fitz CR (1976) Neuroradiology in infants and children. Mosby, St. Louis
2. Pettersson H, Harwood-Nash DC (1982) CT and myelography of the spine and cord. Springer, Berlin Heidelberg New York
3. Post MJD (1980) Radiographic evaluation of the spine. Current advances with emphasis on computed tomography. Masson, New York
4. Genant H (1983) Technical considerations. In: Newton TH, Potts DG (eds) Modern neuroradiology, vol 1. Computed tomography of the spine and spinal cord Chavadel, San Anselmo chap 1
5. Dorwart RH, LaMasters DL, Watanabe TJ (1983) Tumors. In: Newton TH, Potts DG (eds) Modern neuroradiology, vol 1! Computed tomography of the spine and spinal cord. Clavadel, San Anselmo chap 7
6. Kaiser MC, Pettersson H, Harwood-Nash DC, Fitz CR, Armstrong E (1981) A direct coronal CT-mode of the spine in infants and children. AJNR 2:465–466

Vertebral Hemangiomas

D. Reizine, J. D. Laredo, M. C. Riche, J. J. Merland, and M. Bard

The vertebral hemangioma is a vascular malformation giving rise to widely varying clinical pictures. The majority of vertebral hemangiomas remain asymptomatic and are discovered during a post mortem investigation or a routine radiologic examination. Some become apparent through spinal pain or medullary and/or radicular symptoms.

This variation in the clinical picture is explained by the fact that the term vertebral hemangioma embraces many different entities.

Clinical and radiological results, in particular the results of selective angiography allow proposal of a classification for vertebral hemangiomas. This is a subsection of the larger classification of vascular malformations [1].

We distinguish:

1) The asymptomatic vertebral hemangioma, which is intraosseus, of a venous character, nonevolutive.
2) The "pseudotumorous" vertebral hemangioma, which extends beyond the osseous limits; it is of a capillaro-venous nature and evolutive, and has medullary and/or radicular manifestations.
3) Between these two perfectly defined groups, there is the group of vertebral hemangiomas associated with spinal pains. Angiomas remain confined to the intraosseous limits. They can be either venous and nonevolutive or capillaro-venous and evolutive.
4) Lastly vertebral hemangiomas, making up a subsection of complex vascular malformations including Cobb's syndrome and multiple angiomas.

A. Asymptomatic Vertebral Hemangioma

The frequency of macroscopically angiomatous vertebrae that never lead to any clinical signs or symptoms is very high (10% of spines examined in the series of systematic autopsies) [2].

The frequency of asymptomatic vertebral angiomas discovered by chance during a radiologic examination is lower, however. Very small angiomas are not in fact visible radiologically, as shown by x-ray pictures of the anatomic section [3].

Asymptomatic vertebral hemangiomas are a well-defined group with the following characteristics:

It can be seen in clinical practice at all ages

The lumbar spine is the preferred localization: involvement of more than one vertebra is frequent

It is asymptomatic and nonevolutive. It never causes neurologic symptoms

The radiographic appearance is characteristic: Vertical striation or latticed vertebra. The angiomatous process remains localized in the vertebral body, without extension to the pedicle or the rest of the posterior arch. The cortical bone is not affected by any deterioration and there is no extension into the soft tissues.

The angiographic appearance is just as characteristic [4]. There is no anomaly in the arterial or capillary time; pod-shaped opacities may be noted at the level of the vertebral body at the later time, giving the appearance of venous angiodysplasia without extension outside the vertebral body. This group of asymptomatic vertebral hemangiomas must be well individualized: there is no evolutive aspect and invasive investigations are unnecessary.

B. Pseudotumorous Vertebral Hemangioma

This name is reserved for every angiomatous vertebral lesion leading to neurologic symptomatology (medullary and/or radicular) [5–7]. The pseudotumorous vertebral hemangiomas have characteristic clinical and radiographic features: the treatment can be problematic.

I. Physiopathology of the Neurologic Attack

Various associated mechanisms can be responsible for neurologic symptoms.
a) Direct compression of the nervous structures, by an associated epidural angioma is the most frequent mechanism; but direct compression by the augmented volume of the angiomatous bone or, exceptionally, by a hematoma can also occur.
b) A vascular mechanism is also possible: the anterior radiculo medullar artery may be compressed when it begins at the level of the vertebral angioma. Diversion of the blood flow in this case may also be responsible for the neurologic symptoms.

II. Clinical Features

Young adults are preferentially affected, but pseudotumorous vertebral hemangiomas can be encountered at all ages. There is a slight female predominance.

The thoracic spine from T3 to T9 is the predilection site (80%). Lumbar and cervical localizations are rare. The lesion is univertebral, multi vertebral cases are uncommon.

III. Symptoms

The pseudotumorous vertebral hemangioma reveals itself in a medullary compression syndrome of variable onset, which is often progressive over several months but sometimes very sudden.

In 10% of cases paraplegia begins in the last trimester of a pregnancy (Fig. 2). Pain is often mild or even absent. Pseudo-tumorous vertebral hemangiomas revealed by radicular pain are rare and likely to be in the lumbar section of the spine.

IV. Radiologic Features (Figs. 2, 5)

The Standard radiographic appearance of the vertebral hemangioma is characteristic: vertical striation, composed of vertical parallel osseous frameworks of increased density separated by bands of radiotransparency giving a latticework or honeycomb aspect.

Nevertheless there are signs that document the expansive character of pseudotumorous hemangiomas: the angiomatous process occupies the vertebral body and extends to the posterior arch. An extension in to the soft tissues, describing a unilateral or bilateral spindle shapedmass, is frequent (50%).

The osseous cortical borders are puffed up and less well defined than normally. This sign must be looked for when the sides of the vertebral body are rectilinear, or even convex, and in profile particularly at the level of the posterior wall during careful comparison of the angiomatous vertebra with those above and below. The adjacent disk remain intact.

The radiologic aspect of pseudotumorous hemangiomas is rarely ambiguous: it includes corporeal compression and marked osteolysis. Myelography shows a complete block or an extradural medullary compression in relation to the angiomatous vertebra. Two factors associated to a varying degree can be responsible: the tumorous osseous lesion and the epidural angioma.

Selective arteriography must be systematic: the angiographic appearance is characteristic [8, 9]: the angiomatous vertebra is hypervascularized. The arteries supplying the hemangioma are the homologous intercostal arteries, often with recruitment of the over- and/or underlying arteries. The hypervascularization is pathologic (a) in type: the easily visualized arteries of the vertebra have augmented caliber and are tortuous; opacification is rapid,

Fig. 1a–d. Asymptomatic vertebral hemangioma in L2. **a–c** ▷ Standard radiography and tomographies do not reveal any deformation of the osseous contours or any pedicular extension. **d** Arteriography reveals the presence of some pod. shaped opacities at later time

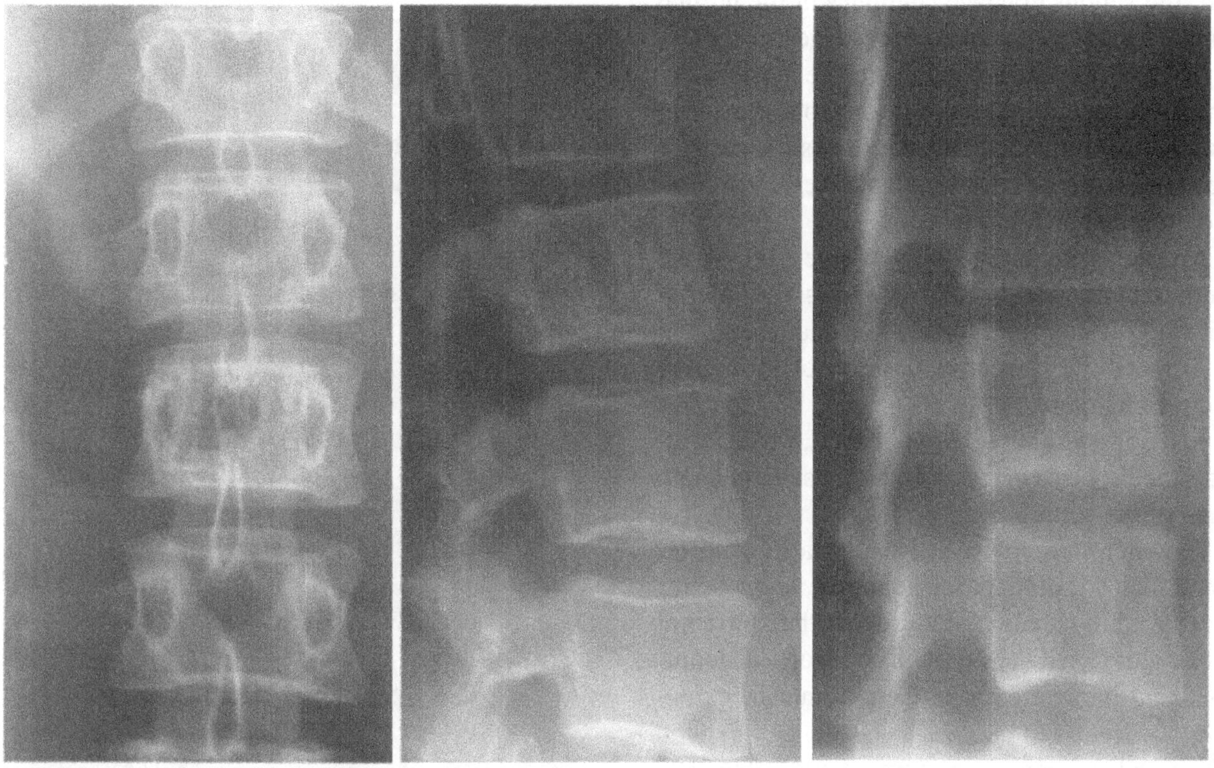

a–c

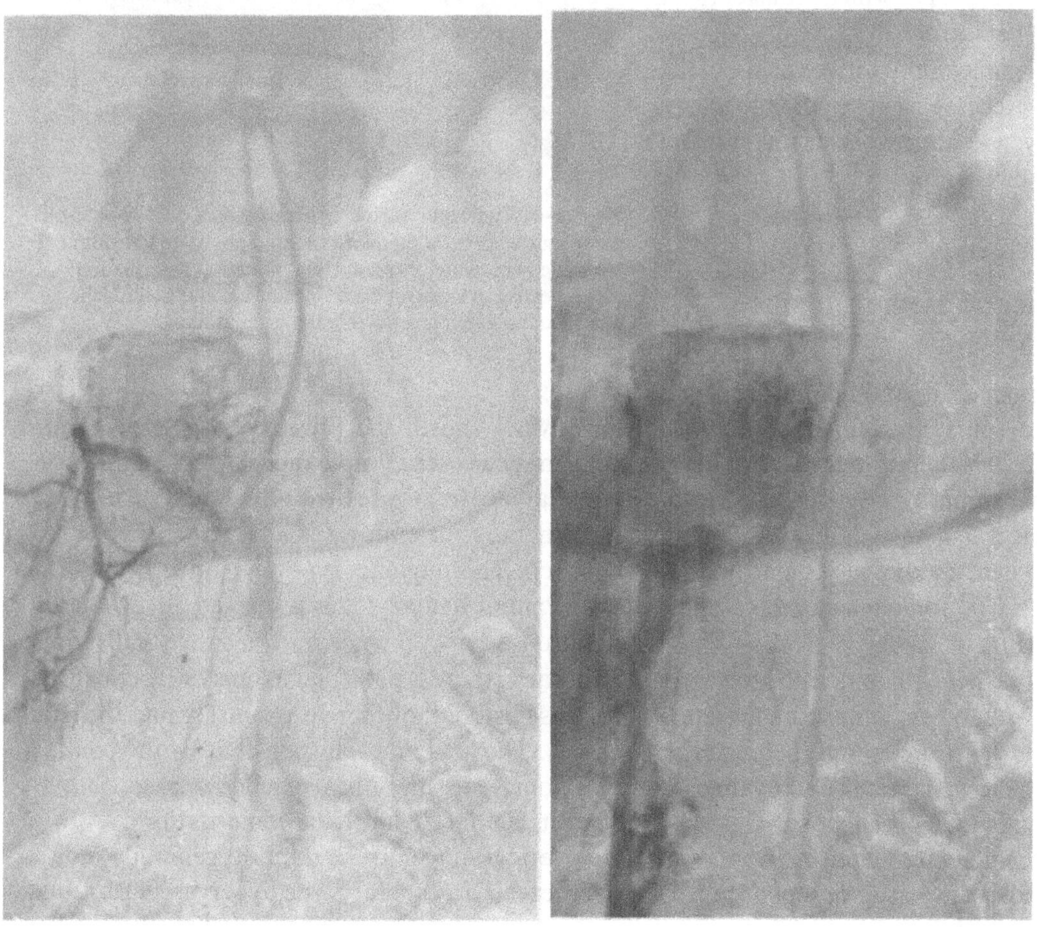

d

homogeneous or heterogeneous and very prolonged: the venous drainage continues in the normal time. This arteriographic aspect suggests capillary angiodysplasia; and (b) in extent: the hypervascularization generally extends throughout the vertebral body and the pedicles, overflows the osseous limits, and extends into the soft paravertebral areas and into the epidural space.

Arteriography is an indispensable part of the pretherapeutic evaluation. It shows the site of origin of the anterior radiculo medullar artery and determines the respective position of this artery and the angioma.

Arteriography allows embolization, which facilitates the surgical operation and can itself attenuate some of the clinical signs.

Tomodensitometry gives greater clarity and precision than conventional radiographs, and a better idea of the extensive nature of the vertebral hemangioma, with blisters and poor cortical definition, and paravertebral and endocanalary extension.

Surgical treatment is performed after preoperative embolization [10, 11], which considerably reduces the risk of hemorrage; it generally consists in decompressive laminectomy with excision of the epidural angioma. Reccurences are possible after a very variable delay, and some workers recommend complementary radiotherapy.

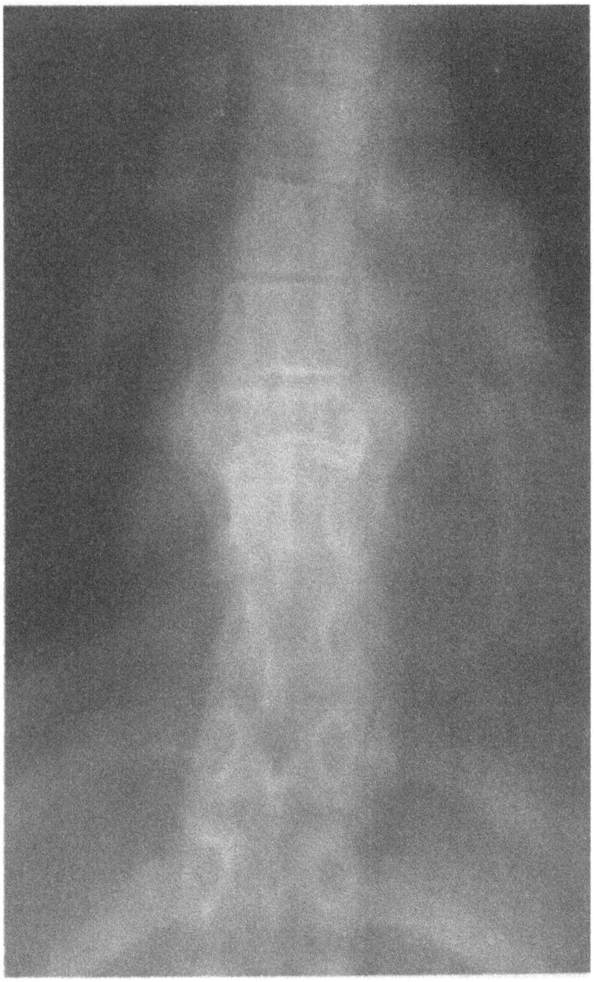

a

Fig. 2a–c. Tumorous vertebral hemangioma in a 30-year-old paraplegic woman. **a** Standard radiography shows angioma at T7, opacity in bilateral spindle, and vertebral deformation; **b, c** Selective arteriography reveals dense and heterogeneous opacification extending beyond the osseous limits

C. Painful Vertebral Hemangiomas

Vertebral hemangiomas are often discovered on a radiograph of the spine prescribed because of isolated spinal pain. It is therefore important to try to classify the hemangioma in the group of nonevolutive venous vertebral hemangiomas or that of evolutive capillary hemangiomas. Standard radiography and, especially, tomodensitometry allow this classification (Fig. 4).

1. Painful vertebral hemangioma is classed as an "asymptomatic" vertebral angioma when the site is lumbar or cervical; the pedicles and the posterior arch are spared; there is no extension to the soft tissues or blistering of the cortical bone.

All other investigations are therefore unnecessary; in fact in our experience arteriography (Fig. 1) has always shown the presence of some venous pods in such cases. Simple radiologic monitoring is necessary. No aggressive treatment (surgery, radiotherapy, or endovascular intervention) must be given. This angioma is not evolutive.

2. Painful hemangioma is classed as a pseudotumorous vertebral angioma when the localization is thoracic; there is pedicular extension; the cortical bone is blistered; or there is extension into the soft tissues. The angioma is responsible for the painful symptoms and must be considered as evolutive since it can have neurologic complications.

Arteriography must be done. It generally shows the presence of capillary type hypervascularization

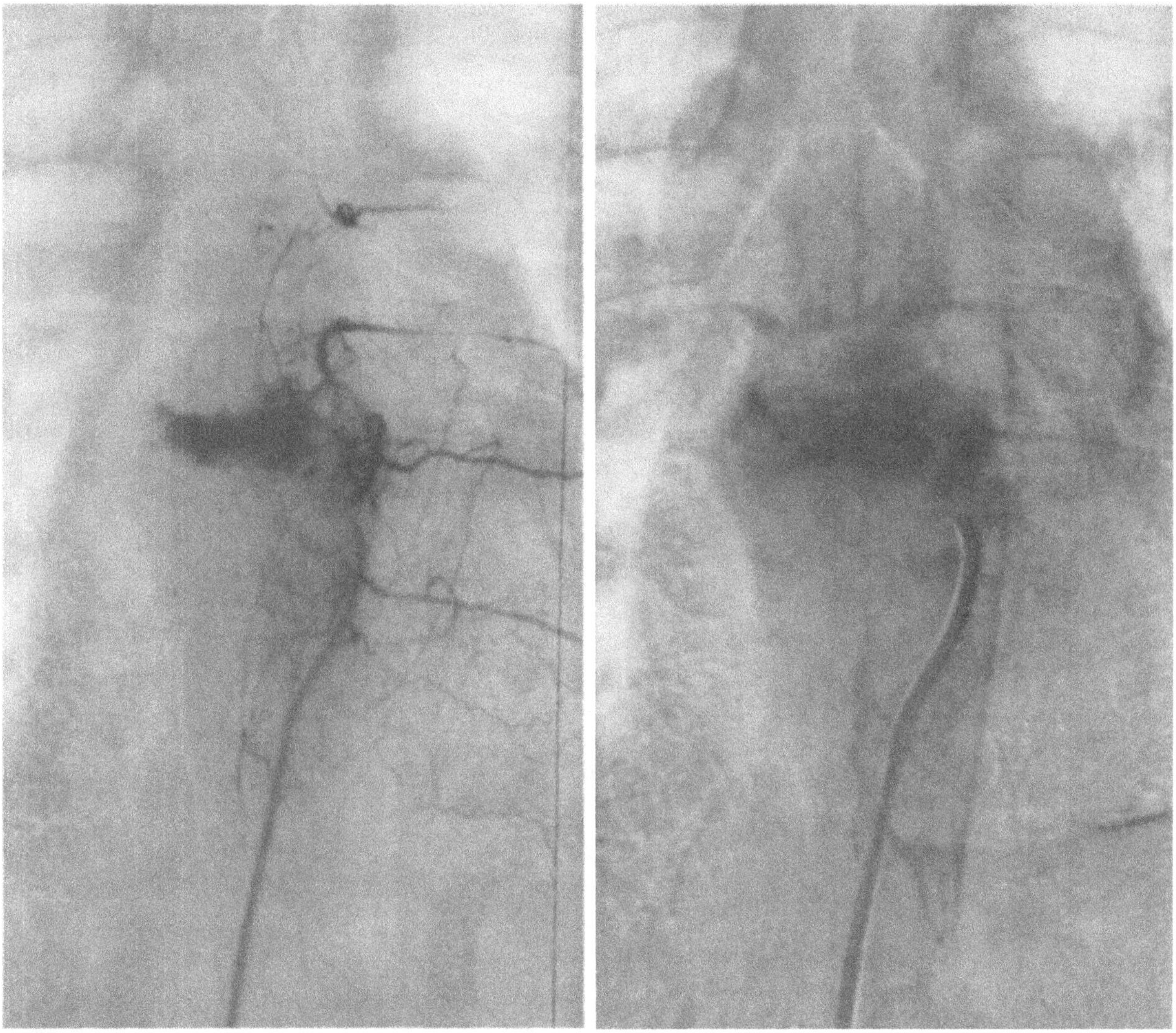

b c

Fig. 2 b,c

similar to that seen in pseudotumorous vertebrae, but without extension into the soft tissues or the epidural space (Fig. 4).

D. Cobb's Syndrome or Metameric Angioma

The osseous angioma is one of the elements of metameric angiomatosis, and is associated with a superficial and/or medullary angioma.

The vertebral angioma is very different: on standart Xray the vertebra is never latticed but rather dense and often the site of a deformation and of large lacunae (intraosseous vascular lacus or erosion due to the angioma of the soft tissues or to a large-volume drainage vein). The arteriographic is also distinctive because it is an arteriovenous angioma of high flow.

The localization can be the thoracic, cervical, or lumbar spine; association with vertebral angiomatosis of a member of the same metamere is also possible. Involvement of more than one vertebra is frequent.

The main symptoms are medullary. This can be due to the medullary angioma, but is often linked with the vertebral angiomatosis, be it by compression or by diversion of the blood flow. The treat-

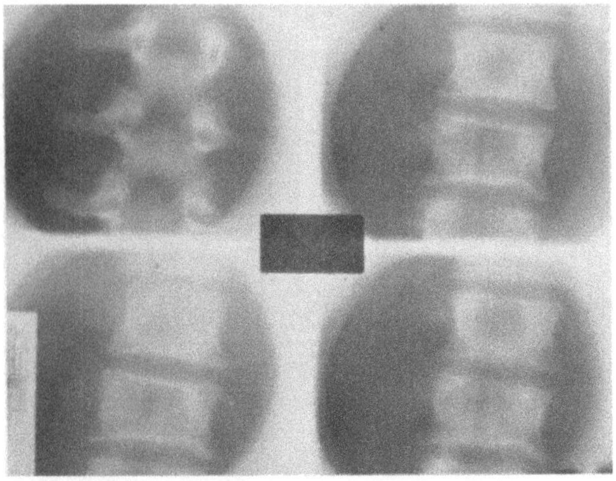
a

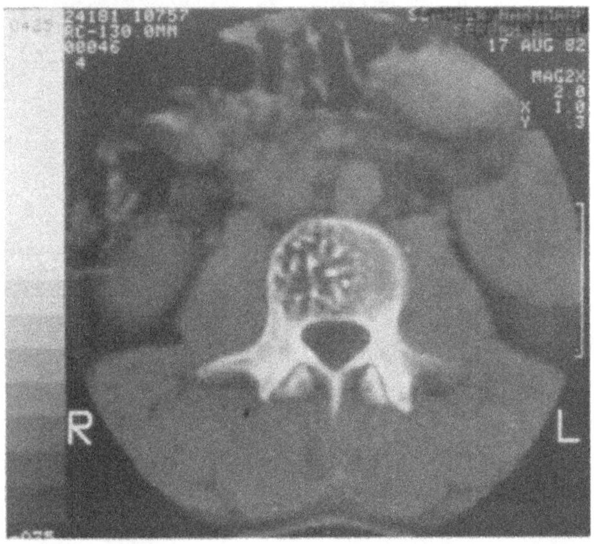

b

Fig. 3a, b. Standart radiographic and TDM appearance of an asymptomatic vertebral hemangioma absence of pedicular and extraosseous extension are easily recognized

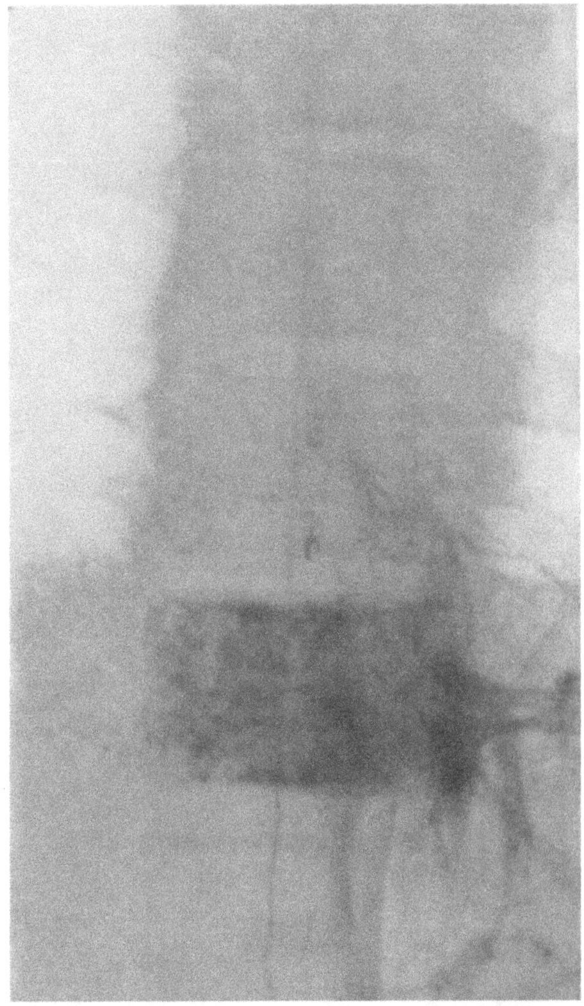
a

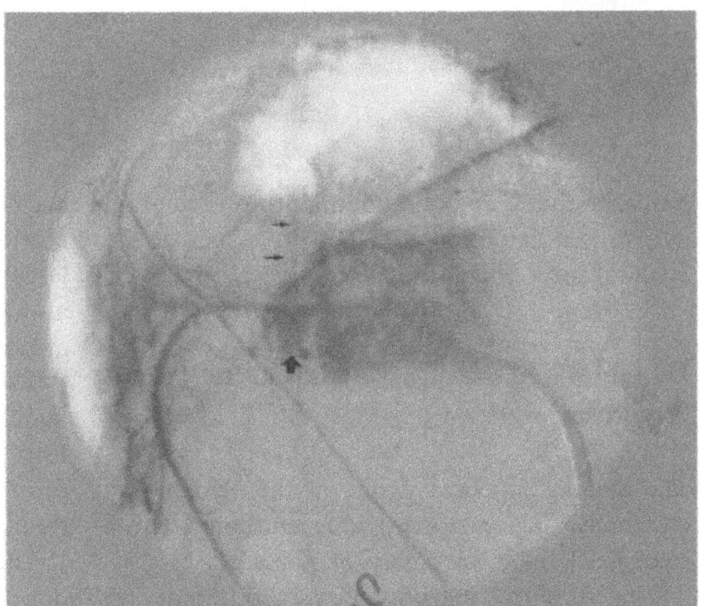
b

Fig. 4 a, b

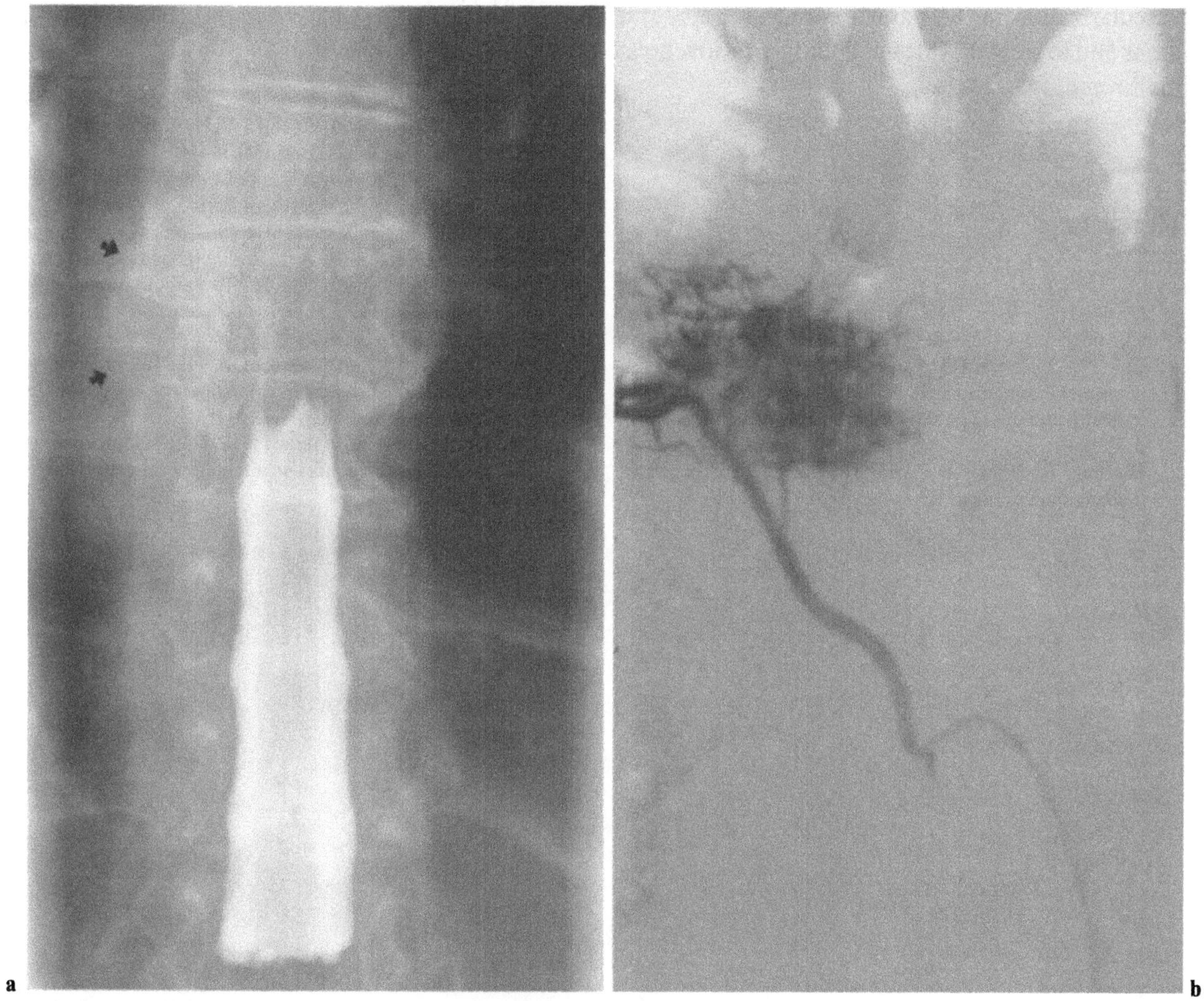

Fig. 5a, b. Tumorous vertebral hemangioma causing progessive paraplegia in a 25-year-old man. **a** Angiomatous vertebra at T5, with extension into the soft tissues: Myelography shows complete block of extradural type; **b** Selective arteriography reveals dense heterogeneous and prolonged opacification of the vertebra

◁ **Fig. 4a, b.** Painful vertebral hemangioma (T8) in a 37-year-old woman with isolated back pain. **a** Selective arteriography revealing hypervascularization of the angiomatous vertebra with pedicular extension; **b** No extension to the soft tissues. Anterior spinal artery is normal *(arrows)*

ment is dominated by embolization. It is the only way of reducing the intense vertebral angiomatous vascularization in the paravertebral and epidural areas and to treat the intramedullary arteriovenous malformation.

References

1. Merland JJ, Riche MC, Monteil J, Hadjean E (1980) Classification actuelle des malformations vasculaires. Ann Chir Plas 25/2:105–111
2. Schmorl G, Junghanns H (1971) In: edn. The human spine in health and disease, 2nd: Grune and Stratton, New York, p 325
3. Sherman R, Wilner D (1961) The roentgen diagnosis of hemangioma of bone. Radiology 86/6:1146–1150
4. Djindjian R, Merland JJ (1981) Angiography of the spinal cord and spinal tumors. Springer, Berlin Heidelberg New York p 140–160
5. Virinder M, Gupta, E, Tuli D (1980) Symptomatic vertebral hemangiomas. Clin Radiol 31:575–579
6. Bergstrand A, Hook O (1975) Vertebral haemangiomas compressing the spinal cord. Acta Neurol Scand 39/1:60–64
7. McAlister UL, Kendall BE, Bull SWD (1975) Symptomatic vertebral haemangiomas. Brain 98:71–80
8. Reizine D (1981) Angiographie des tumeurs primitives du rachis. Dissertation, University of Paris
9. Manelfe C, Djindjian R (1977) Exploration angiographique des angiomes vertébraux. Acta Radiol [Diagn] 13:820–825
10. Lepoire J, Montaut J, Picard L (1973) Embolisation préalable à l'exérese d'un hémangiome du rachis dorsal. Neurochirurgie 19/2:173–181
11. Benati A, Da Pian R, Maschio A (1974) Preoperative embolisation of a vertebral haemangioma compressing the spinal cord. Neuroradiology 7:181–183
12. Djindjian R, Hurth M, Houdart R (1971) Angiomes médullaires dysplasies vasculaires segmentaires ou generalisées. Rev Neurol 124:121

Metastatic Disease of the Spine and Spinal Canal

M. LEMORT, L. DIVANO, and L. JEANMART

Since the spine is one of the most frequent localizations of secondary neoplasms affecting bones or causing neurologic disorders, it is of outstanding importance to have a good perception of the wide variety of radiologic appearances this form of disease can have.

Some published work [15, 19, 30, 32, 42, 43] has treated this subject, presenting important features discovered by conventional radiologic examination, i.e., plain radiographs, conventional tomography, and myelography. Primary importance also attaches to isotopic studies of the skeleton for screening of bone lesions [12].

However, rapidly developing new technique, particularly computed tomography (CT) and, more recently, nuclear magnetic resonance (NMR) are providing the physician with new tools for diagnosing complications in the cancer patient. In the particular field of spinal metastases, CT provides an accurate method for appreciating tumoral spread toward paravertebral soft tissues and, of course, the vertebral canal. When performed after intrathecal injection of water-soluble contrast media it can reveal small epidural infiltrations, which can be difficult to see with conventional myelography. Relations with paraspinal tumoral masses can also be demonstrated. There is no doubt that when further clinical evaluation has been accomplished NMR will be even more efficient for this purpose, and will perhaps prove more highly specific.

Regardless of these new technique, isotopic studies and conventional radiology remain the basic methods for detecting, characterizing, and evaluating bone metastases (treated in different ways).

Other methods (CT in our experience) must be considered as second-line technique for the resolution of specific diagnostic problems.

The aim of this chapter is to give a brief statement of the clinical significance of metastatic disease of the spine, to give some clues to understanding of its origin, and above all, to illustrate radiologic aspects of the disease examined both by "conventional" techniques and by CT.

Since epidural metastases have most frequently (up to 85%) [36] proved to be associated with vertebral involvement at the same level, and the dissemination pathways frequently seem to be the same, it seems logical to discuss spinal bone metastases and epidural metastases as a nosologic entity. Leptomeningeal involvement and intramedullary metastases, however, are local expressions of a generalized involvement of the CNS in most cases. Spinal metastatic arachnoiditis will be briefly reviewed here, but intramedullary metastases, which are generally associated with brain metastases, have been discussed by Baleriaux (this volume).

A. Frequency

According to all statistics, metastatic tumors account for the great majority of tumors of the skeleton in general [36, 41], and particularly of the spine [11]. The clinical significance of osseous metastases is considerable. About 15%–30% of deaths investigated by autopsy are due to osseous metastatic involvement [42]. It is not exceptional that pain linked with the secondary osseous involvement, particularly collapse of an infiltrated vertebra gives rise to the first symptoms of neoplastic disease.

The frequency of osseous involvement and its localization vary according to the nature of the primary tumor. Most metastatic tumors are carcinomas [37], the most frequent sites being the breast, the prostate, the lung, the thyroid, the kidney, and then the digestive tract [8, 36, 37]. Melanomas and sarcomas also often metastasize to bone. If we consider the distribution by sex, in woman cancer of the breast is responsible for nearly 70% of osseous metastases; in men, cancer of the prostate is responsible for nearly 60% and cancer of the lung for 25% [42].

In some series, lymphomas and multiple myelomas are significant origins of metastases [9, 16].

Of the primary tumors responsible for vertebral metastatic involvement, 33% are tumors of the breast and 28% are tumors of the lung, followed by tumors of the digestive tract and of the prostate [35]. Different authors record different proportions, according to the recruiment procedures. In the spine, the area most frequently affected by metastatic lesions is the thoracic section [3, 8, 36, 37], followed by the lumbar section [37]. If we consider the vertebrae individually, the 5th lumbar vertebra is the single one most often involved [14]. Metastases from cancer of the prostate have a particular predilection for the sacrum and the lumbar spine (59% lumbar involvement; 85% sacral and pelvic involvement) [42]. The same is true for other pelvic primary tumors (uterus, rectum) [4].

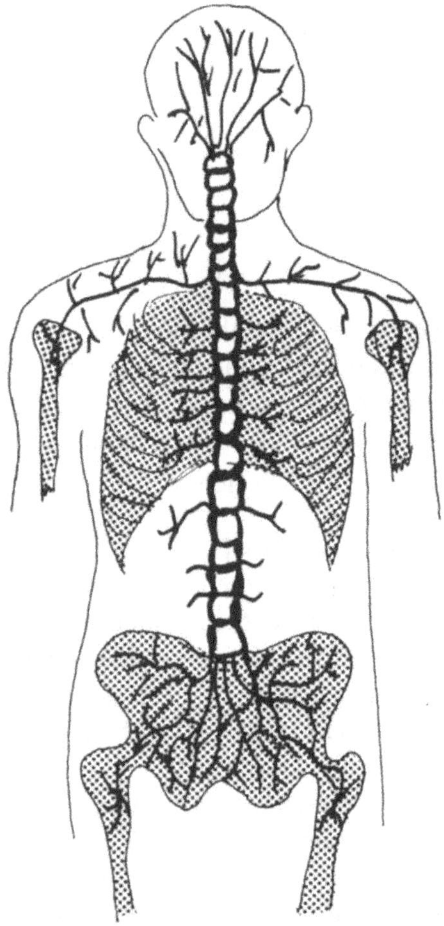

Fig. 1. Schematic of the vertebral venous plexuses and of their anastomotic relations with the peripheral venous networks. (After BATSON [5–7])

B. Dissemination Pathways

Examination of dissemination pathways of the tumor cells from the primary site toward the vertebral column allows a better understanding of a phenomenon which must be appreciated in a dynamic way and not as the result of a random distribution.

In 1940, Batson [5–7] pointed out the role of the vertebral venous plexus in metastatic spread. Made up of veins with thin, valveless walls, the plexus behaves as a vast venous reservoir in which the direction of flow is variable. Contracting multiple anastomoses both with the vena cava system at every level and with the superficial veins of the trunk and the roots of the limbs, the deep cervical veins, and the cranial veins, it is itself a system (cf. Fig. 1) with the capacity (dependent on variations in flow) for transporting neoplastic cells and emboli while bypassing the heart and the pulmonary filter, which explains the cases of "paradoxical" dissemination, where osseous metastatic involvement occurs in isolation and no other organs are found to be affected at autopsy. Batson's work, taken up and expanded by other researchers [2, 10], shows evidence of a passage of flux towards the vertebral network on abdominal compression. Abrams, in his angiographic studies in vivo of the vertebral and azygous system however, noted frequent opacification of this plexus even in the absence of any abdominal compression [1]. It is nevertheless easy to imagine that any modification of abdominal or thoracic pressure associated with a change of position, with coughing, or with Valsalva's experiment can favorize the passage of neoplastic emboli via the vertebral venous system.

The plexuses considered to be left over from the embryonal plexiform venous system [1] are made up of the perivertebral venous network, of the peridural network, and of veins draining the vertebral bodies (basivertebral veins).

All these elements are largely anastomosed among themselves. These anatomic particularities account for the high frequency of the osseous infiltrations at the same level as an epidural lesion.

The role of the vertebral venous system offers a satisfactory explanation for the preferred vertebral localization of osseous metastases, the preferred lumbar topography of metastases from pelvic neoplasms, and the involvement of osseous sites in the absence of pulmonary localization, but cannot explain everything about dissemination. So, it is surprising to discover that while osseous metastases from prostate cancers are frequent, other pelvic neoplasms (bladder, ovary, uterus), although as stated above they occur preferentially at the lumbosacral level, nevertheless have only a low propensity to metastasize to bone.

The arterial route is also certainly responsible for some neoplastic embolizations at the osseous level, but its role in the involvement of the spine is very probably less important than that of the vertebral venous system [22]. On the other hand, as at the cerebral level, it plays a primary role in metastasis to medullary localizations.

The lymphatic tract seems less important here, although occasional cases of infiltration from that origin cannot be excluded; however, the possibility of neoplastic emboli passing from the lymphatic system towards the venous system suggests again that cancer cells reach the bones or the peridural spaces by way of this venous system.

The cerebrospinal fluid is a classic route of dissemination in the case of cerebral primary tumors: it is involved in the cerebral metastasis of extraneural cancers which have broken through the cortex or the ventricular walls and provoked carcinomatous meningitis. This type of dissemination is followed by the appearance of carcinomatous arachnoiditits and of multiple disease sites in the marrow and in the roots of the cauda equina. Extension of an epidural lesion to the meningeal layer is rare, the dura mater presenting exceptional resistance to infiltration by neoplastic tissue [31]. However, subdural infiltration owing to contiguity is occasionally seen [8].

Finally, the last mechanisms to be cited are gradual local extension, particularly starting from paravertebral adenopathies with secondary osseous infiltration of the vertebra, and canal infiltration by way of the intervertebral foramen. Lymphomas frequently metastasize by this last route [27, 39].

C. Radiological Patterns of Bone Metastases of the Spine

Conventional radiology is the first examination, after isotope studies, for detecting and monitoring bone metastases. Plain radiographs of the entire spine are part of the standardized examination of the skeleton, based upon statistical distribution of metastatic lesions. In our experience [12], this includes examination of the entire axial skeleton with femurs and humeri.

Classic patterns of metastatic bone infiltration are described as destructive (lytic) lesions, densifying (blastic) lesions, and mixed lesions, where both types of changes are associated in varying proportions. These patterns are not fixed, nor is any of them specific for a particular primary tumor [25].

Some tumors more frequently cause certain types of changes [42] but these characters are inconsistent. Prostatic neoplasms, for instance, are known often to give rise to densifying metastases (Fig. 2); lung cancer, to destructive lesions (Fig. 8), and breast cancer to mixed-type lesions; variability is great, however. In the same patient, and even in the same bone, purely lytic and purely blastic lesions can be found at the same time. These characters can also change over time, with the effect of treatment.

A lytic process has multiple causal factors. The pressure effect of the tumor growing inside the bone and ischemic necrosis surrounding the bony lesion are definitely important. Osteoclasts are also concerned, essentially in the earlier stages. A large body of experimental evidence indicates that bone resorption-activating substances produced either by tumor or by bone tissue reacting to tumor vicinity, are partially responsible for the lytic phenomenon, either directly, or by stimulating osteoclastic activity. Prostaglandins (essentially PGE 2) and prostaglandin-like substances, produced in larger amounts by tumoral breast tissue than by normal breast tissue, may favorize a lytic process.

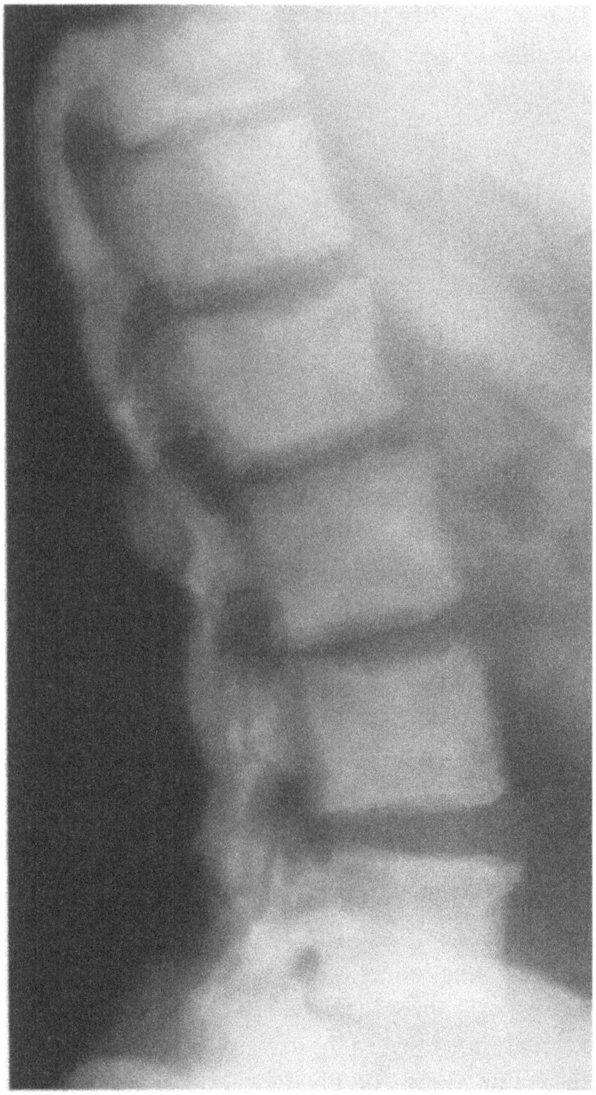

Fig. 2. Metastasis of a prostatic cancer. The lateral projection shows diffuse densifying metastatic infiltration of the entire lumbar spine

The collagenolytic action of neoplastic breast tissue can be enhanced by estrogens produced by tumor or host. An osteoclastic activation factor (OAF) is produced in large amounts by tumors of the hematopoietic system and seems of paramount importance in the osteolytic changes encountered with these tumors.

Therefore, it is obvious that the specific biologic activity of cancer cells will greatly influence their inclination to settle and develop in an osseous environment and will modulate the morphologic expression of bone metastases.

Osteoblastic changes are a response of the osteogenic bone tissue to the vicinity of tumoral tissue. There is a relationship between the speed of the tumoral growth and the osteoblastic response: very slow-growing metastases may be totally densified, without any lytic area.

Finally, the appearance of densified areas during treatment may reflect a healing process and not a worsening of the metastatic disease [26] (Fig. 3). Conversely, a new lytic lesion developing during treatment must be considered as an indication of an unfavorable course, as also must the disappearance of a dense healed area, which can give a false impression of a normalizing plain radiograph (Fig. 4).

In some cases, however, with sufficiently long-term survival, complete restitution of the normal macroscopical aspect of bone can be observed, with disappearance of sclerotic changes either after treatment or even spontaneously [33] (Fig. 3).

It is obvious that a purely lytic metastasis appears in the radiographic image at a much later stage than a mixed or osteoblastic metastasis. As long as there is no cortical disruption, even an extensive lytic lesion of a vertebral body can remain mute on standard radiographs and even on conventional tomography, especially if the vertebra is osteoporotic and if the linear sweep is used, in which case the effacement shadows can mask weak density gradients. The excellent spatial and densitometric resolution of the CT examination, particularly when it is associated with high-resolution programs, allows clear demonstration of such a lesion.

This examination is therefore indicated when an isotopic scan is positive at a given level and conventional radiology is negative or doubtful [20, 23, 34] (cf. Fig. 4).

Generally, an osteoblastic or mixed metastasis will be clearly seen on the standard radiogram. Some small lesions can be missed, however, particularly in the event of superpositions, and in case of doubt recourse to tomography or CT can be useful (Fig. 5).

Diffuse condensation of a vertebra ("ivory-like" vertebra) can be revealed, but not very frequently (cf. Fig. 6).

When the metastatic lesions induce cortical disruption, increased vertebral fragility frequently leads to deformations corresponding to pathologic a 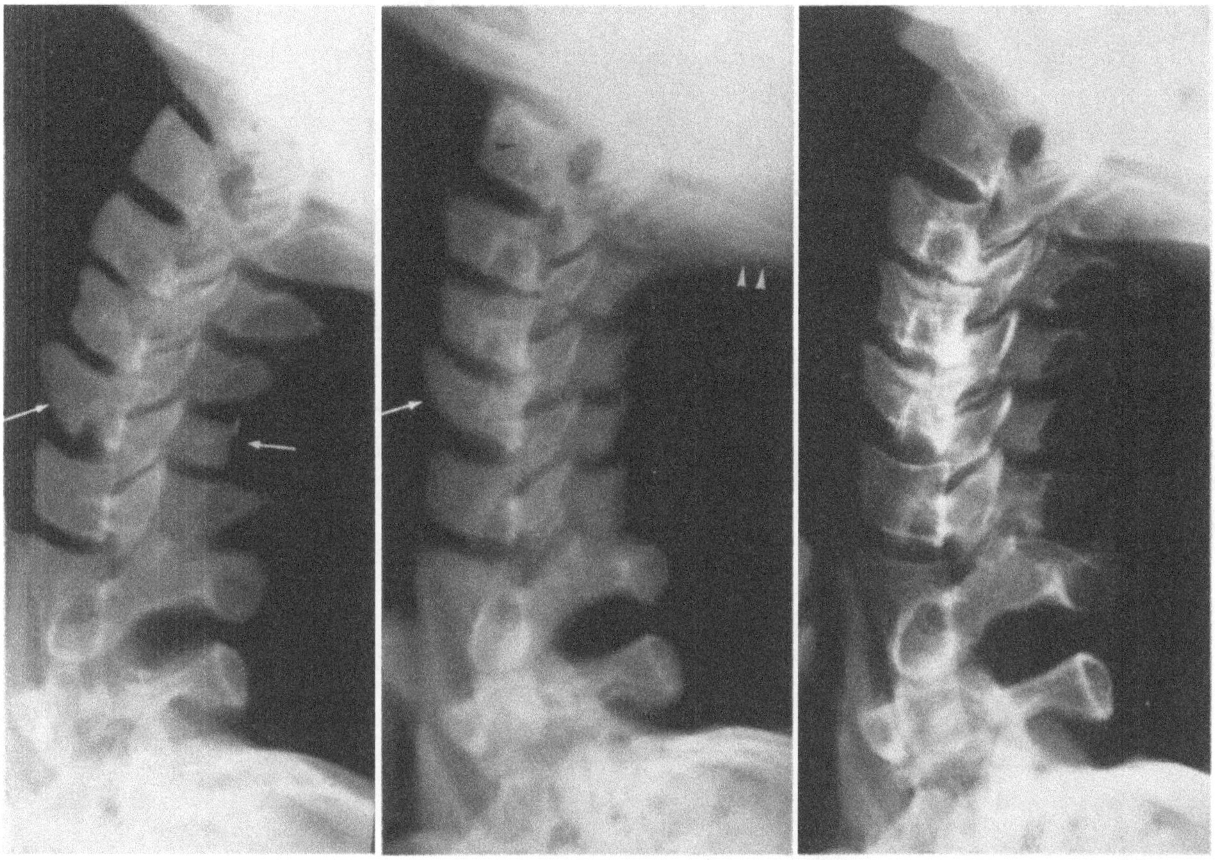 b, c

Fig. 3a–c. Evolution over 18 months of metastasis from a cancer of the breast to the cervical spine, with favorable response to hormonochemotherapy. **a** Initial status (August 1981): Lytic lesions of the vertebral body and the spinous process of C4 (*arrow*) and other vertebral bodies showing discrete diffuse heterogenesis. The spinous of process C7 does not appear to be altered. **b** After 4 months of treatment, collapse of the anterior part of the vertebral body (*arrow*) has occured, while the spinous process of the same vertebra is trending to reminaralize. Areas of osteocondensation are appearing at the vertebral body level and in the spinous process of C7 (*arrowheads*). **c** Toward normalization of the osseous stroma at the level of C7 (January 1983)

fractures (Fig. 7). A vertebral collapse can be the first sign of the metastatic illness, and even of the neoplastic illnes.

The pedicular involvement frequently described as characteristic of vertebral metastatic infiltration is by no means mandatory. Its absence is not an argument against metastatic infiltration of the spine. Numerous vertebrae can be massively invaded (at the level of vertebral bodies) without any pedicular anomalies. With 83% vertebral body involvement, Sellwood [32] warns of 29% pedicular involvement. It is true, however, that the disappearance of a pedicle (showing up as an image of a "one-eyed" vertebra; (Fig. 8) or the isolated condensation of a pedicle (Fig. 9) strongly suggests vertebral metastatic infiltration. Vertebral bodies and pedicles are not the only vertebral regions that the radiologist must observe carefully. The lysis of a transverse process (Fig. 8) or of a spinous process can arise in isolation and cause painful symptoms or an isotopic hypercaptation. Finally, neoplastic tissue, having disrupted the cortical bone, can extend beyond the limits of the vertebra and into the paravertebral soft tissue, showing a "spindle-like" image on conventional examinations (Fig. 7). This image was encountered by Sellwood [32] in 15% of cases of osseous metastasis to the vertebral column. Examination by CT is useful in such cases for specifying extension of the tumor to the soft tissues.

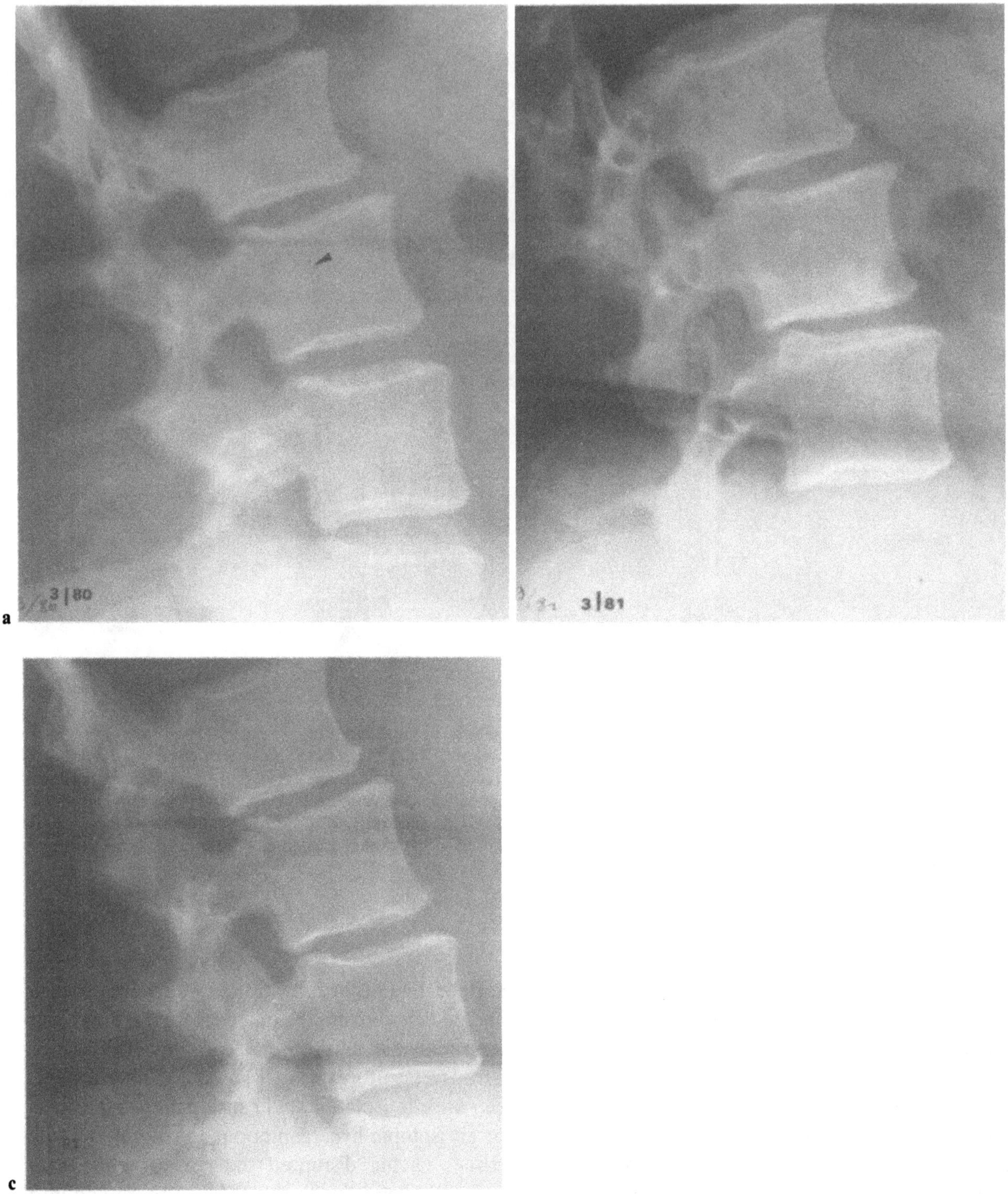

a b c

Fig. 4a–e. Evolution of metastatic infiltration from a breast cancer, with known osseous generalization, which stabilized during treatment (March 1980). **a** Bone sclerosis (*arrowhead*); after 1 year (**b**) and 21 months (**c**) of treatment this has virtually disappeared; an appearance of "normalization" is achieved. In June 82 (**d** standard tomography) metastasis at the level of L2 is patent, with lateral collapse of the vertebral body. **e** CT examination carried out in December 1981, when the standard radiograph appeared virtually normal, gives good visualization of the lytic infiltration area outlined by a border of osteosclerosis. This metastasis is thus seen to have densified during treatment, which has led to development of the lytic character, ultimately causing vertebral deformation. During the course there was an apparent phase of paradoxical normalization of standard x-ray films

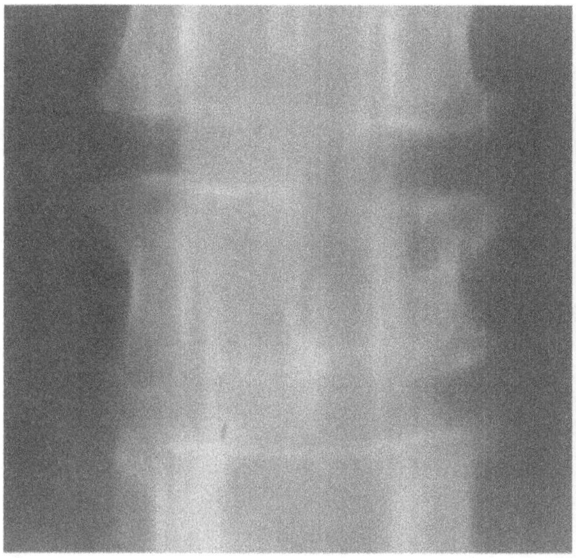

d

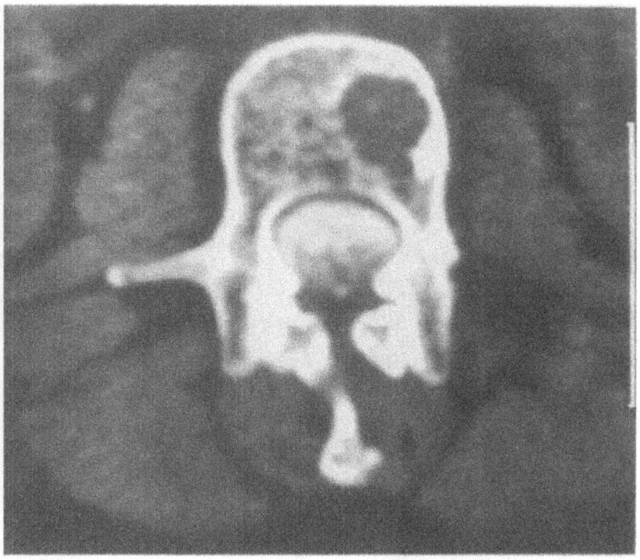

e

Fig. 4 d, e

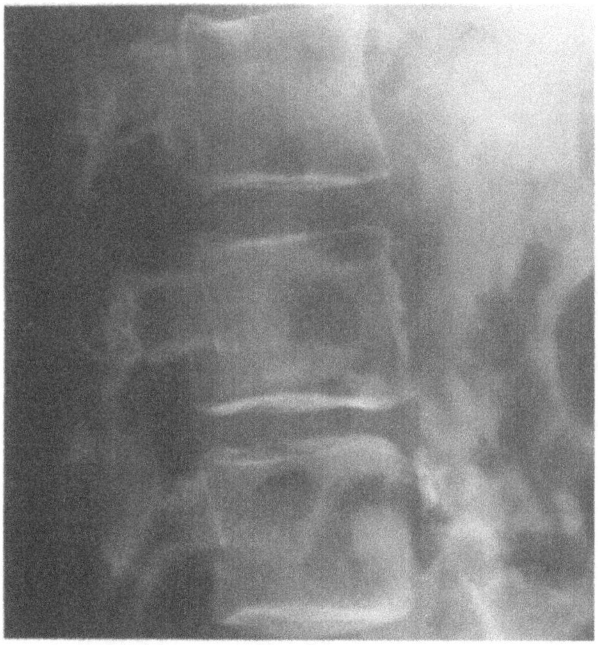

a

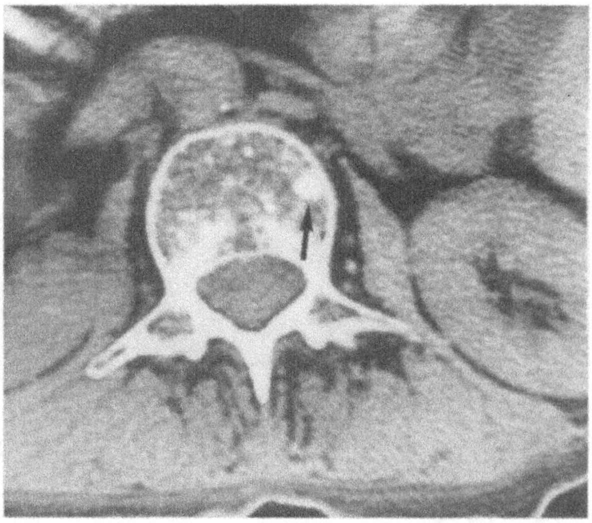

b

Fig. 5 a, b. Metastasis from a breast cancer. Standard x-ray of the spine (**a**) does not show an unequivocal image of metastatic infiltration, because of significant superpositions. High-resolution CT of L3 (**b**) shows diffuse infiltration by small blastic lesions (*arrow*); three vertebrae (L2–L4) are affected. Considered invidually, an image of this kind can correspond to a benign condensing islet. The multiplicity of these images at the level of the three vertebral bodies examined indicates the metastatic nature in this case

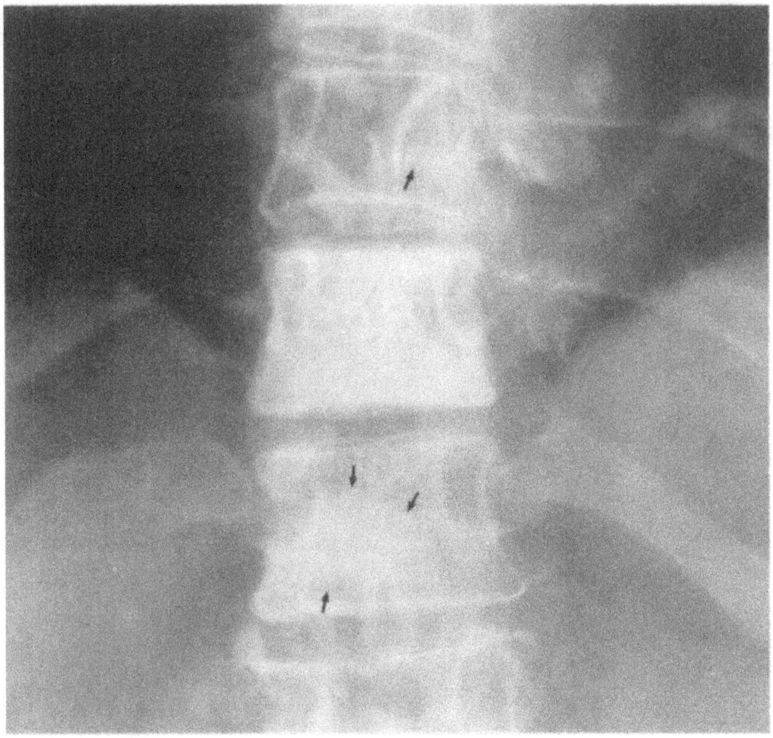

Fig. 6. Metastasis from a breast cancer. Standard x-ray shows a typical image of ivory vertebra at the level of T10. Note also the presence of irregular areas of densifying changes in the adjacent vertebral bodies (*arrows*)

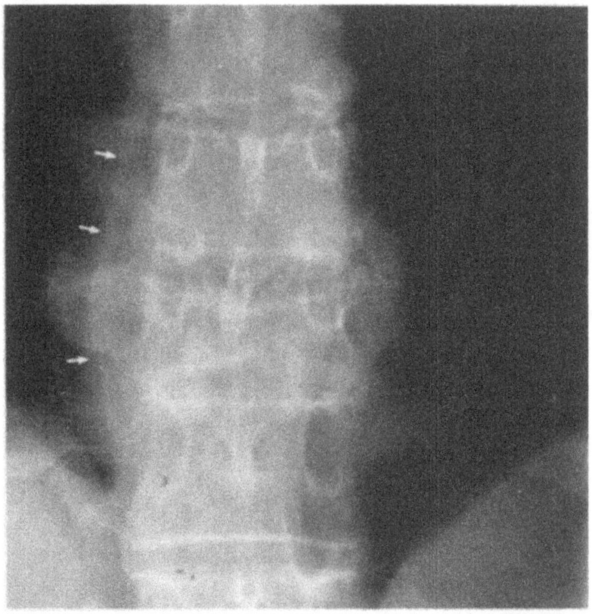

Fig. 7. Metastasis from a breast cancer. Isolated vertebral collapse was the first manifestation of generalized osseous involvement. Note also the existence of a paravertebral soft tissue "spindle" (*white arrows*)

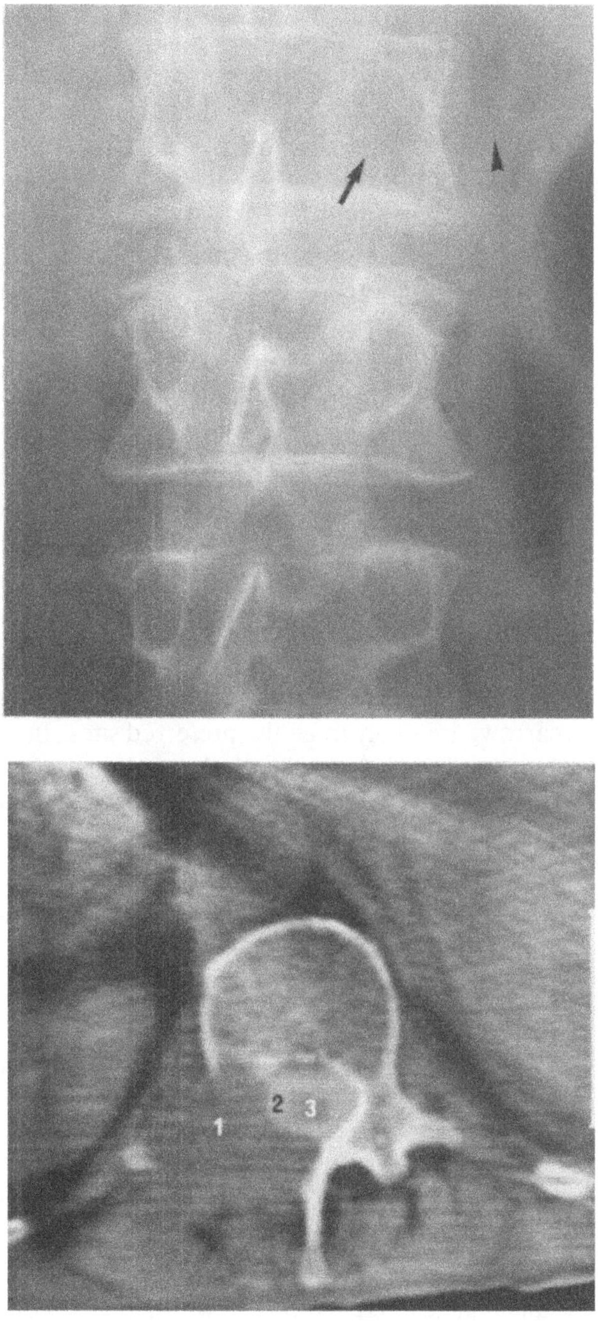

a

b

Fig. 8a, b. Metastasis from a lung cancer. Standard radiograph (**a**) reveals disappearance of the left pedicle of L1 (*arrow*) and of the left transverse process (*arrowhead*). CT examination (**b**) performed after myelography with water-soluble contrast medium, shows that the tumoral tissue (*1*) has totally destroyed the left pedicle and the lamina of L1, and virtually all of the transverse process. Overflowing towards the spinal canal the tumor comes in contact with the opacified dural sac (*2*) at the level of the conus medullaris (*3*) (epidural metastasis)

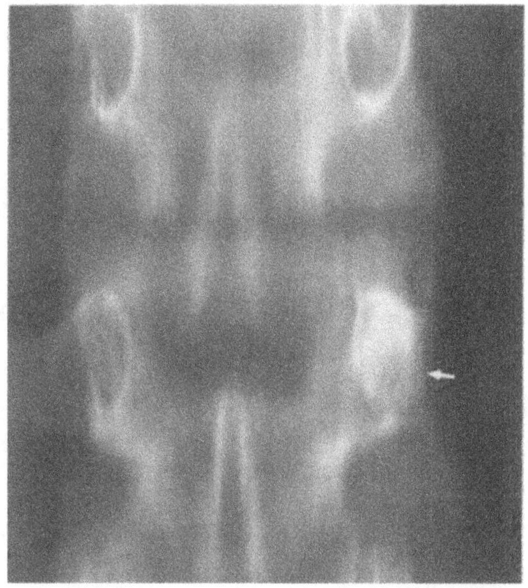

Fig. 9. Metastasis from a breast cancer. Tomography (linear sweep) shows isolated condensation of the left pedicle of L2 (*arrow*)

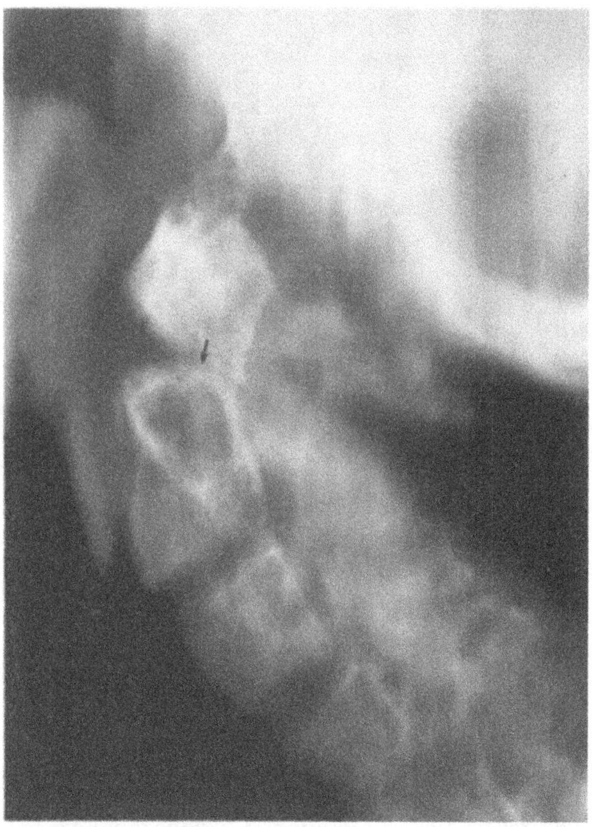

Fig. 10. Metastasis from a breast cancer. Tomography (linear sweep) reveals infiltration of mixed type of the ondotoid process of C2 with pathologic fracture (*arrow*)

a

b

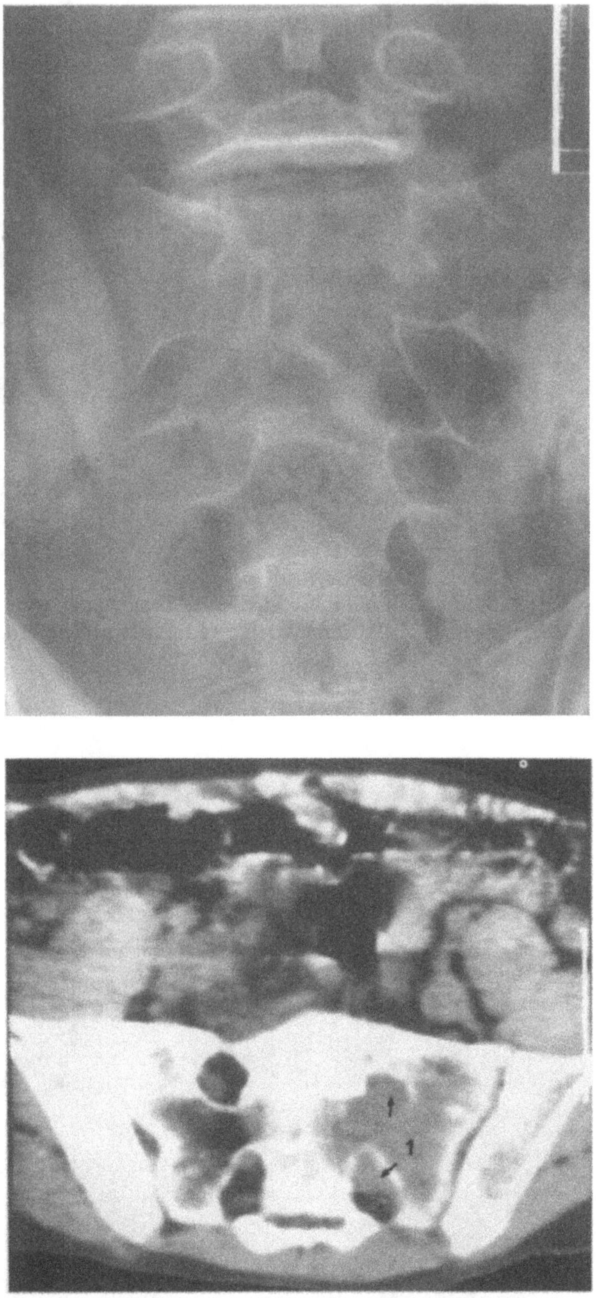

Fig. 11 a, b. Metastasis from Ewing's sarcoma. Standard radiograph (**a**) shows a discretely less dense aspect of the left part of the sacrum, which however is difficult to verify because of the superpositions. CT (**b**) reveals a large infiltration of the left part of the sacrum by metastatic tissue (*1*), with infiltration of the adjacent sacral foramina (*arrows*). There was also presacral infiltration at a lower level

The area of the cervico-occipital junction requires particular attention. The consequences of an untreated infiltration at this level can be extremely serious, particularly if a pathologic fracture (Fig. 10) occurs. A CT examination of the area must be undertaken on the slightest suspicion.

Infiltration of the sacrum, when discrete, can sometimes be difficult to assess on a standard radiograph, on account of frequent superposition of parts of the digestive tract. When there is any suspicion of sacral involvement, a CT examination is extremely useful. In addition to the osseous lesions, it can demonstrate extension to the presacral area and invasion of the sacral intervertebral foramina, which is responsible for radicular attacks (Fig. 11).

In multiple myeloma, bone lesions take on the aspect of an osteolytic phenomenon involving the entire skeleton except for the base of the skull. The frequency of spinal lesions explains the frequency of paraplegia in this disease. In the Waldenström series (130 cases) [40] the most frequently involved vertebra were the last thoracic and first lumbar, which is inconsistent with the hypothesis that the 4th and 5th lumbar vertebrae, being richer in bone marrow, are likely to be the preferred sites. In the Onofrio series [29] the cervical vertebrae and the first thoracic vertebra are rarely involved. On the other hand, thoracic vertebrae lower than T3 are frequently involved. Odelberg-Johnson [28] has described three typical types of myeloma from the aspect of radiologic appearance (Fig. 12):

Well-circumscribed osteolytic lesions
Plurilobular conglomerates of cystic rarefaction, resembling clusters of soap bubbles
Osteoporotic-type lesions

The most common radiologic picture is that of an osteolytic lesion, sometimes widely destructive, sometimes finely defined. The problems in differential diagnosis are concerned with senile osteoporosis, which however, rarely involves the cranial vault and the extremities; with lymphomatous infiltration; or with metastasis from solid tumors: Jacobson et al. [21] report in this connection how rarely pedicular involvement occurs with myeloma.

In childhood leukemia the radiologic appearance consists in diffuse demineralization, sometimes with horizontal radiolucent bands at the upper and lower limits of the vertebral body, as can be observed in other osseous localizations, especially

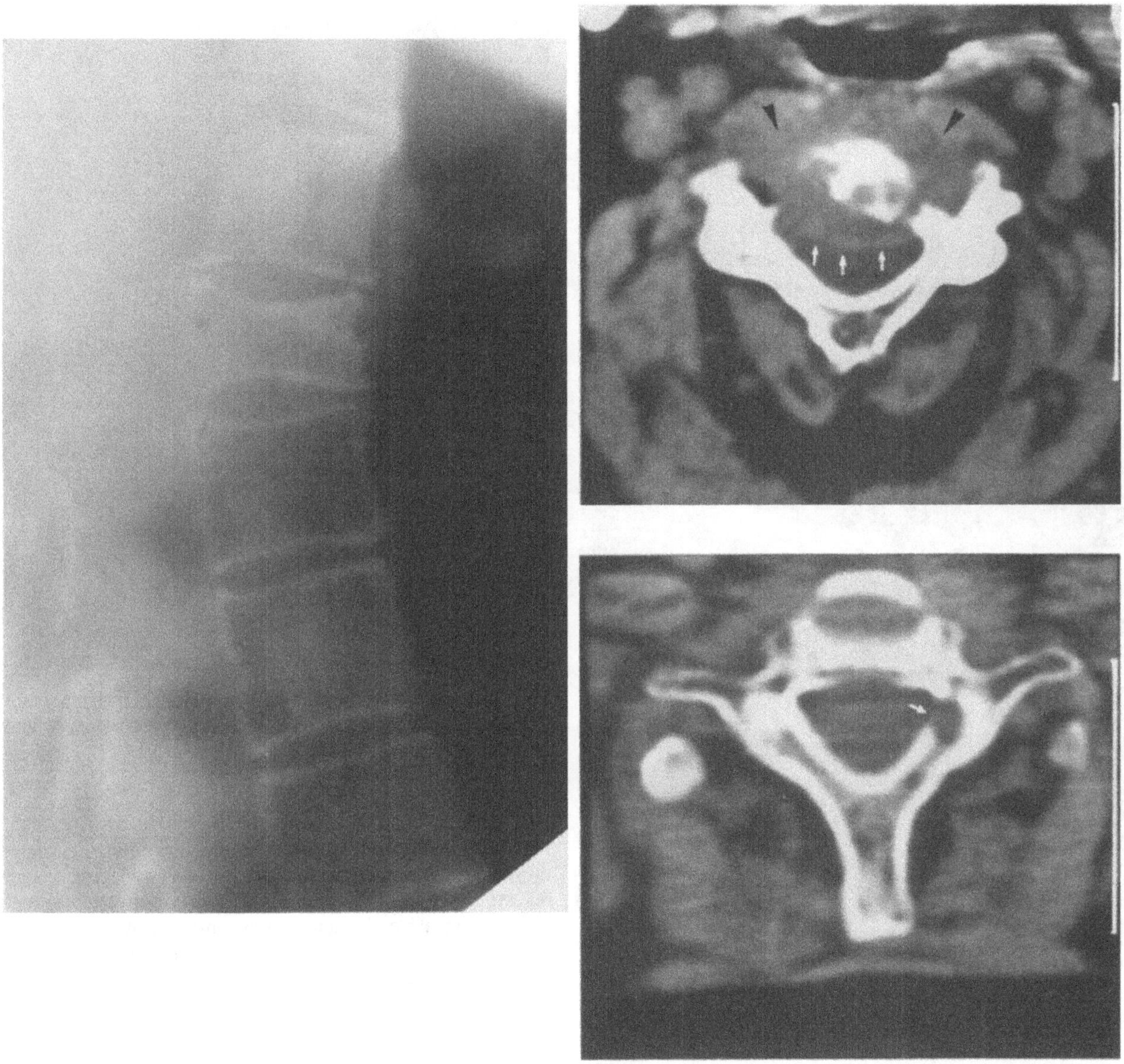

a b c

Fig. 12. a Multiple myeloma, with diffuse osteoporotic-type infiltration, of the thoracic spine. Note the collapse of a mid-thoracic vertebra, giving a diabolo form. (Courtesy of Dr. Laissy, Service Professor Nahum, Hôpital Beaujon)
b, c Infiltration of the cervical spine by multiple myeloma: **b** CT in addition to virtually complete lysis of C3 by the myelomatous lesion, reveals protrusion of tumor tissue into the peridural spaces (*arrows*) of the vertebral canal and into the prevertebral muscles (*arrowheads*); **c** at the level of C7 there are small finely defined lytic lesions, notably at the level of the posterior arch, where there is cortical effraction (*arrow*). These small lesions were not detectable on conventional x-rays

at the metaphyses of long bones. Localized zones of osseous destruction and even osteosclerotic reshaping can be observed in acute leukemias [43].

In adults, the radiologic aspect is that of diffuse demineralization, which could cause vertebral collapse. However, in adult acute leukemia death frequently occurs before the osseous involvements can be visualized radiologically.

The osseous lesions caused by Hodgkin's disease, lymphosarcomas, and reticulosarcomas are similar in appearance and difficult to differentiate radiologically. Purely osteolytic, mixed and osteosclerotic lesions are found. In the presence of lymphomatous disease, a purely lytic aspect (Fig. 13) suggests lymphosarcoma; on the other hand, an osteosclerotic or mixed aspect is more suggestive of Hodgkin's disease (Fig. 14). A particular feature of lymphomas is the possibility of secondary vertebral lesions originating from the paravertebral lymphomatous masses (involved lymph nodes), causing

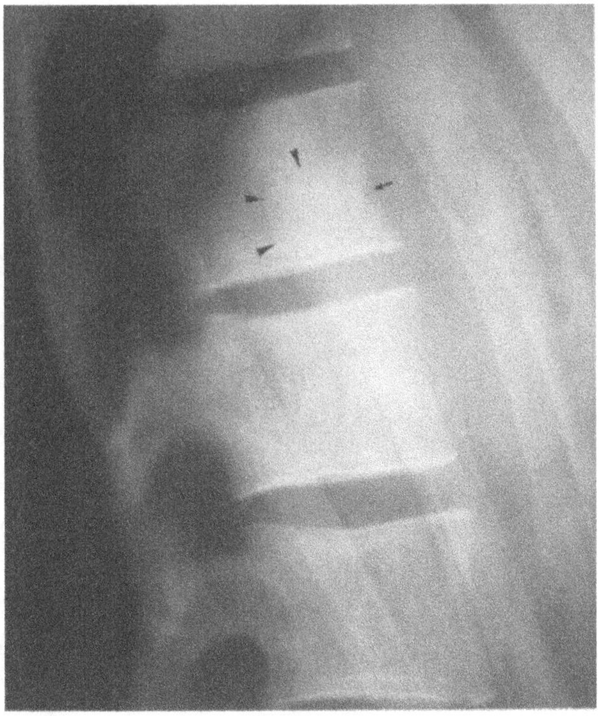

Fig. 13. Vertebral infiltration by a non-Hodgkin's lymphoma. The lesions are mixed in type, with lytic predominance and multiple vertebral collapse

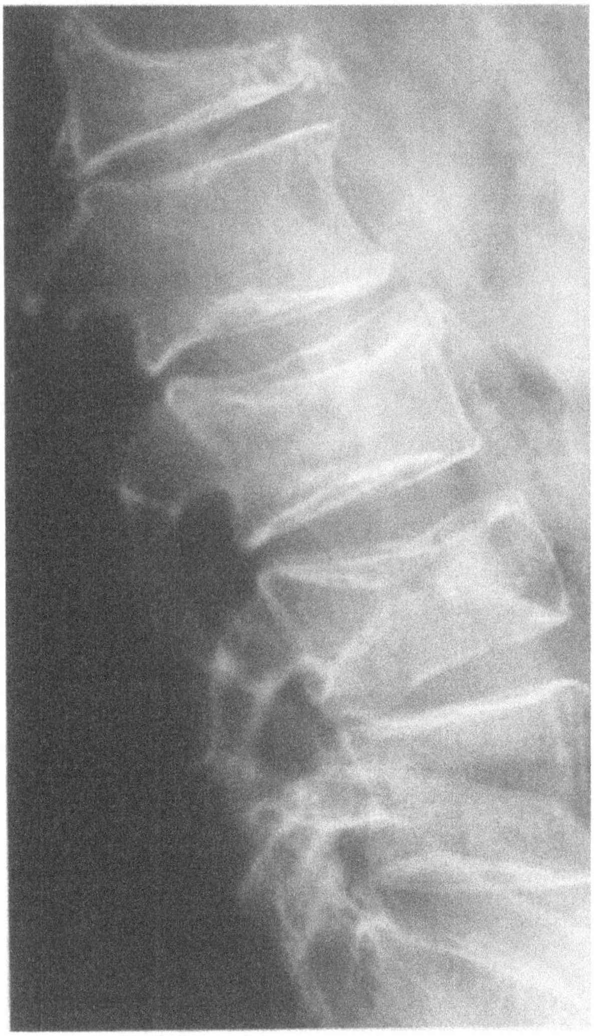

Fig. 14. Hodgkin's disease. In addition to the diffuse densification of L1 (*1*), we note an anterior erosion (scalloping, gouge defect; *arrow*) at T12, originating from a perivertebral and retroperitoneal lymphomatous mass confirmed by CT. Note the osteosclerotic reaction at the periphery (*arrowheads*) at the level of the vertebral body

curvilinear erosions ("gouge" defects or scalloping) [43] (Fig. 14) of the anterior part of the vertebral body, associated with an osteosclerotic reaction of the adjacent area. This kind of lesion can be seen in lymphosarcomas and chronic lymphoid leukemias, but the metastatic nodes of solid tumors occasionally have this appearance [43]. Scalloping is also found in the presence of aortic aneurysms or tuberculous abscesses, but without alterations of the adjacent bone structure.

D. Radiological Signs of Intracanalar Lesions

The clinical consequences of epidural neoplastic infiltration are always serious and can take the form of an acute neurologic deterioration leading to paraplegia in a few hours. The development of an expanding process inside a closed space causes rapidly compressive phenomena at the medullary level, with edema of the nervous tissue and impairment of the vascular supply [38]. The lesions can rapidly become irreversible, and early detection of the epidural infiltration is imperative to increase the chances of success of any treatment.

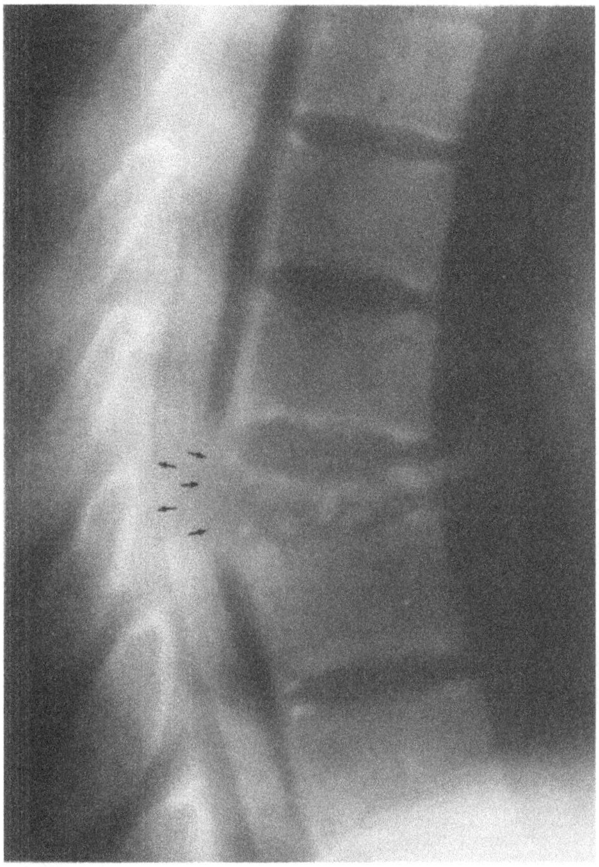

Fig. 15

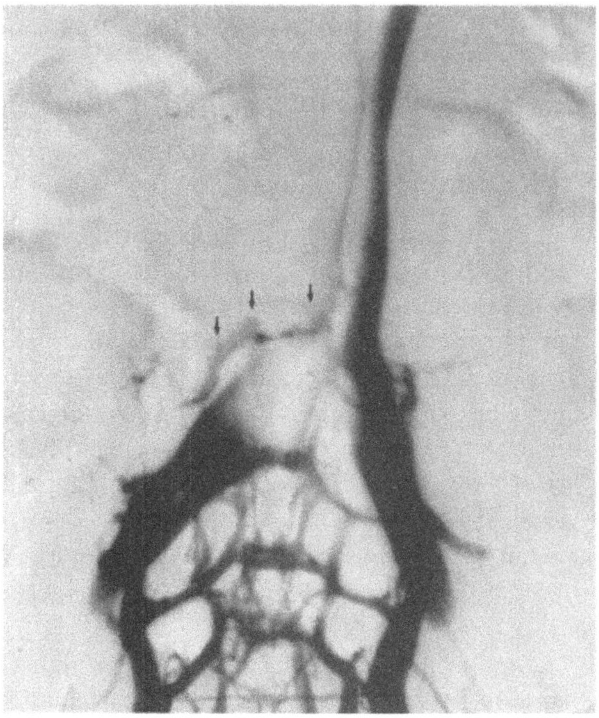

Fig. 16

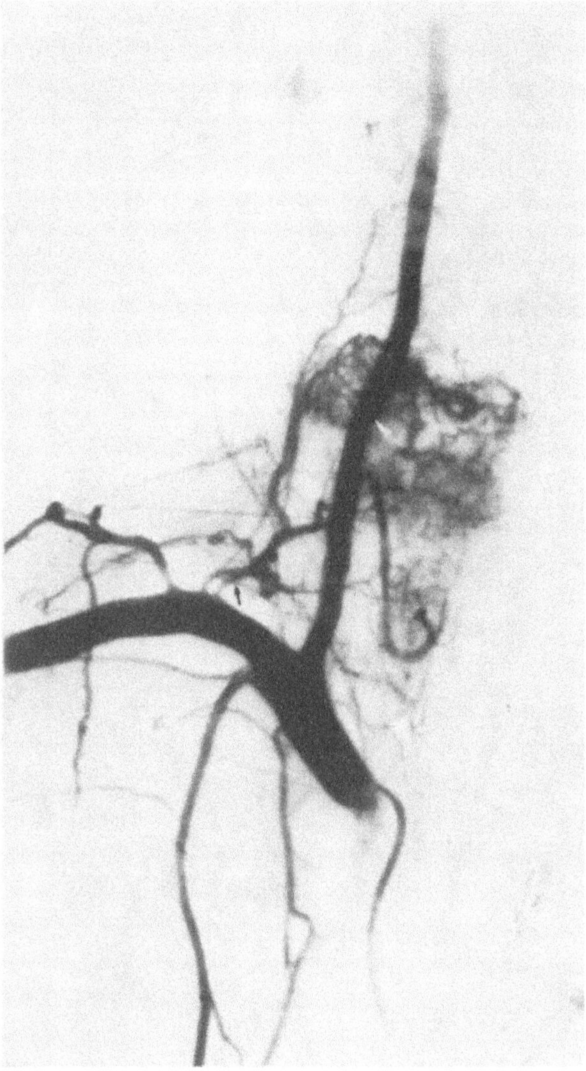

Fig. 17

Fig. 15. Metastasis from an undifferentiated carcinoma. Gas myelography shows anterior medullary compression and lytic osseous infiltration of T9 spreading toward the peridural spaces. Note the loss of anterior and posterior perimedullary images (*arrows*). (Courtesy of Dr. Théron and Dr. Burguet, Caën)

Fig. 16. Carcinomatous epiduritis (undifferentiated malignant tumor) in a 5-year-old child. Phlebography shows an epidural block at L3 (*arrows*), indicating the inferior pole of the infiltration which, at surgery, was found to extend down to T11. (Courtesy of Dr. Laissy, Service Professor Nahum, Hôpital Beaujon)

Fig. 17. Metastasis from a clear cell renal carcinoma. Arteriography (catheterization of right subclavian artery) shows tumorous "blush" at the level of C7 and T1, vascularized by a deep cervical collateral of the right subclavian artery (*arrow*) and displacing the vertebral artery (*arrowhead*)

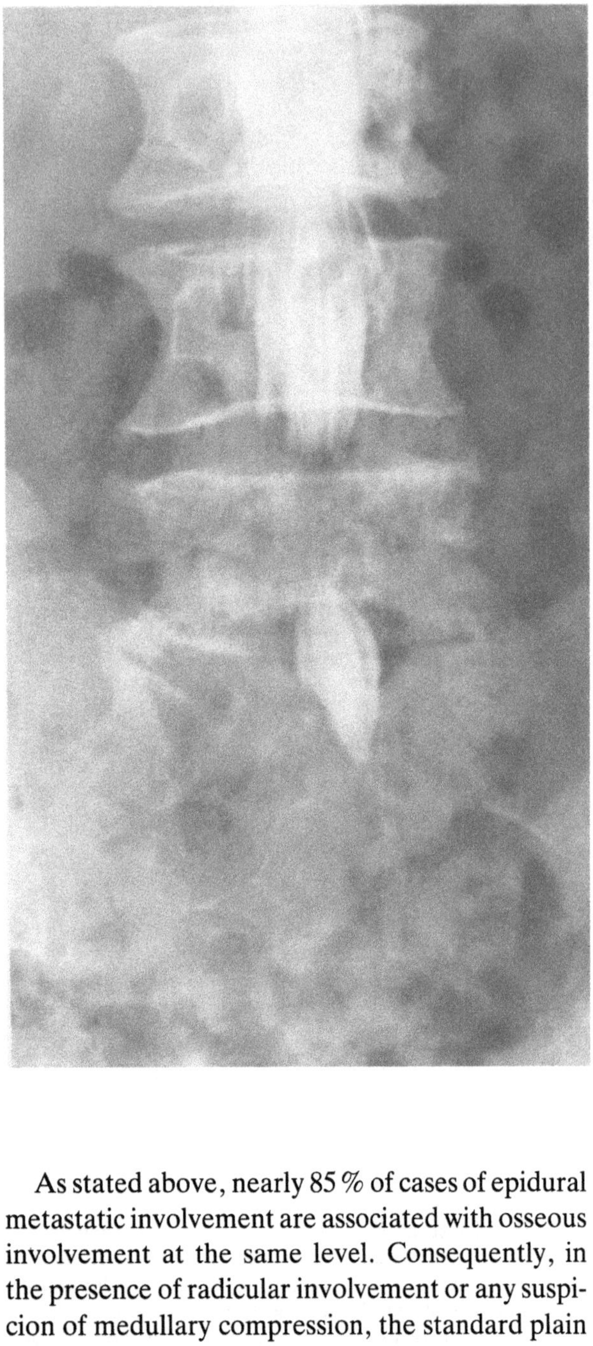

a

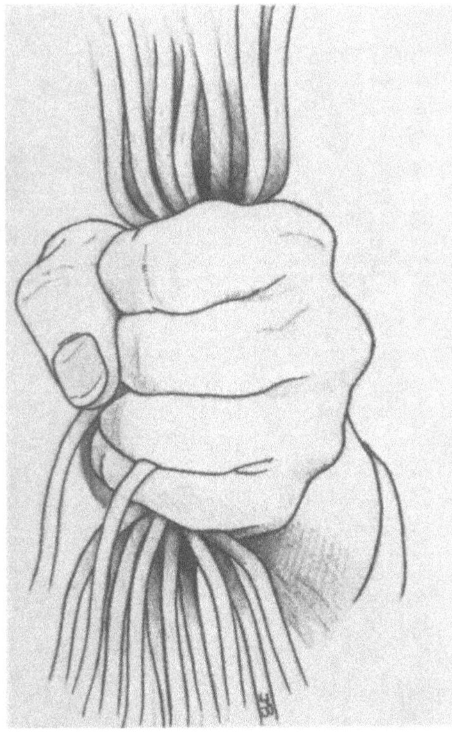

b

Fig. 18a, b. Metastasis from a breast cancer. Myelography (**a**) shows epidural infiltration with subtotal myelographic block at the level of L5, itself involved by an osseous infiltration of mixed type. Note the characteristic appearance of the compression of the dural sac and the roots ("sheaf in hand" image: **b**) with fragmented appearance of the superior border contours

As stated above, nearly 85% of cases of epidural metastatic involvement are associated with osseous involvement at the same level. Consequently, in the presence of radicular involvement or any suspicion of medullary compression, the standard plain radiograph of the spine must be examined with the greatest care to detect the slightest sign of osseous infiltration at this level. The posterior arch must be examined as carefully as the vertebral body; the size of a small lesion of the posterior arch could be out of all proportion to that of the associated intercanalary lesion [15]. Evidence of an osseous infiltration at the level suspected on the grounds of a clinical examination is in itself highly suggestive of an epidural metastasis. Myelography and CT will generally only confirm the diagnosis. Conversely, radiologic detection of vertebral osseous metastasis must be extended to include a careful neurologic examination for definitive detection of any discrete sign of radicular involvement or medullary compression. LONGEVAL et al. [24] point out the frequency (50%) of positive myelographic examination in patients presenting with vertebral osseous metastasis but with no signs of medullary compression: two of these patients (3.5%) did not even show any signs of radicular attack.

Consequently, there must obviously be no hesitation in performing a myelographic examination without delay, preferably associated with computed myelography, on the slightest clinical suspicion (especially with discrete signs of radicular attack). We cannot, however, consider systematic performance of myelography in all asymptomatic patients who may have vertebral metastases, because a negative result of this examination does not exclude the possibility of later epidural involvement. The use of nonabsorbed lipidic products, although allowing by simple tip over, confirmation of the persistence or the removal of a block, is not compatible with the fine detection of small incipient lesions, and it compromises later CT examination by reason of artefacts produced.

The myelographic examination inconstestably constitutes the most reliable means of detection of epidural infiltration. In our experience, this examination is best practiced with aqueous contrast medium (solution of metrizamide with concentration of 250 mg I/ml) and followed almost always by CT examination. The aqueous medium is selected because it gives a sharp image and is compatible with the CT examination. A manometric measurement systematically precedes the injection, which is monitored under scopic control (see KAISER and CAPESIUS, this volume). Other techniques, such as gas myelography (Fig. 15) and phlebography (Figs. 16 and 17), also allow the identification of epidural infiltration and precise determination of the effects either on the spinal cord or on the peridural venous network (KAISER and CAPESIUS, this volume). Recourse to CT centered on the clinically and/or myelographically suggestive level is justified by the better detection of very small lesions and sharper delimitation of the extension, and in some cases it makes up without loss of efficiency for myelographs whose technical quality has proved unsatisfactory: the properties of the water-soluble contrast agent, particularly its rapid dilution, cause a rapid loss of diagnostic efficacy if the slightest technical hitch occurs during the examination. The densitometric sensitivity of the CT examination allows the maintenance of satisfactory opacification eben if the contrast medium is no longer discernable in standard radiology.

The most typical myelographic image indicating epiduritis is an indentation or lamination varying in degree, of the opaque column. Sheathing of the dural pouch can be complete, giving rise at the lumbar level to the "sheaf in hand" image (Fig. 18).

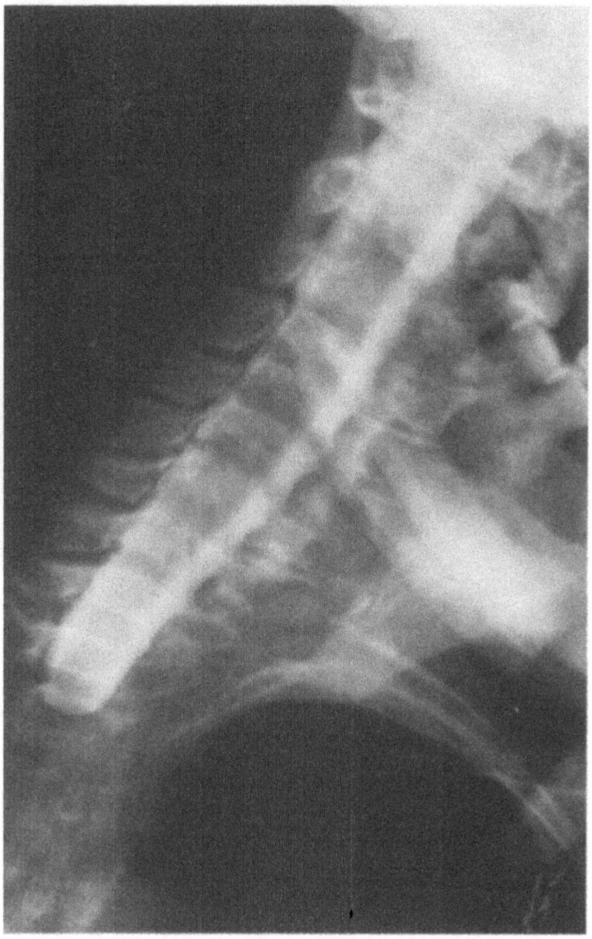

Fig. 19. Metastasis from a breast cancer. Myelography with contrast injection by the upper route (laterocervical) shows a complete block due to epiduritis at the level of T3.
Note the regular borders of the opaque column at the level of the block

The degree of compression of the dural pouch determines the appearance of a complete or partial block. In the cases of a block due to epiduritis, the margins of the opaque column are generally described as irregular and indented (Fig. 18). This is not always found (Fig. 19). When the lower myelographic block is complete and it is necessary to know the exact extent of the process, a second intrathecal injection of contrast medium by the upper (laterocervical or suboccipital) route allows definition of the superior limit of the lesion (Fig. 19). The possibility of multiple lesions at different levels must not be ignored, however. A seemingly total myelographic block can in reality be subtotal and associated with a certain passage of contrast medium, though insufficient to give an upstream

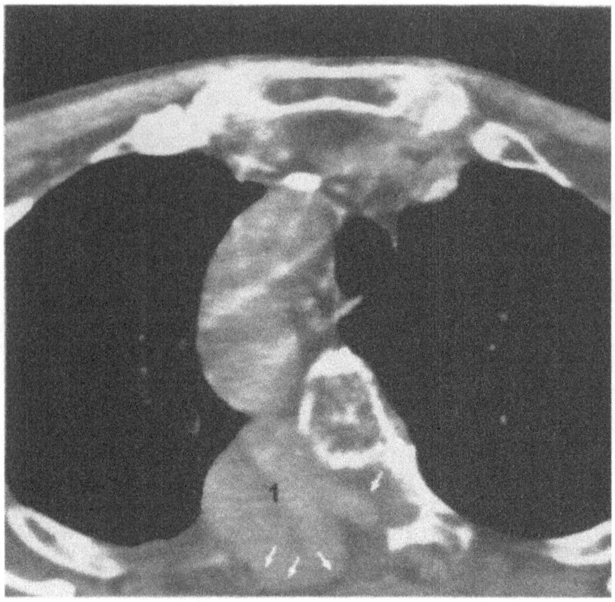

b

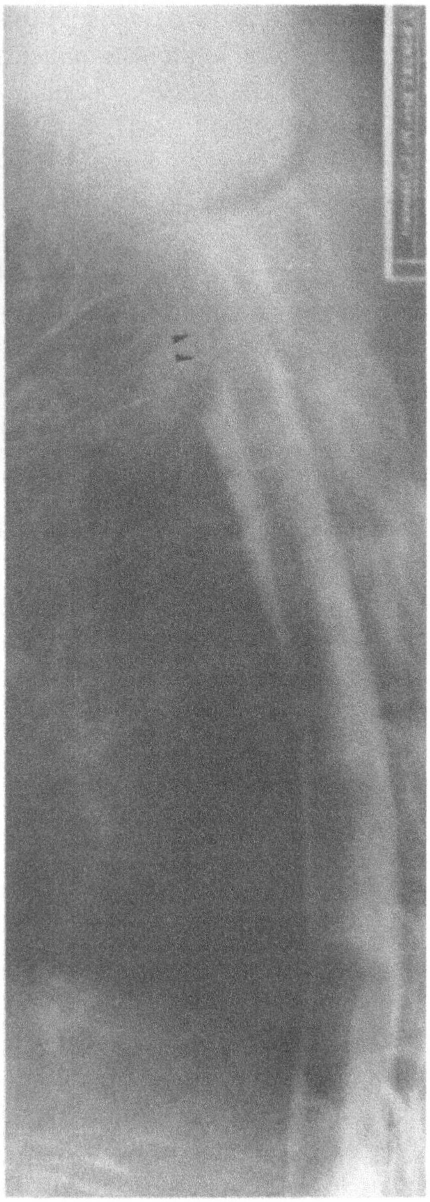

a

Fig. 20a, b. Metastasis from a lung cancer. Myelography with contrast injection by the lower route (**a**) shows appearance of a complete block at a high thoracic level (*arrowheads*) CT (**b**) allows precise determination of the major spread of the tumor mass (*1*) towards the paravertebral soft tissues (*arrows*), and also allows visualization of persistent passage of the metrizamide (*arrow*) into the dural sac encompassed by the epiduritic process. The passage of contrast medium was adequate for appreciation of the superior limits of the lesion and for study of the cervical spine by CT myelography

contrast; in this case CT allows detection of such areas of poor opacification and precise determination of the superior limit of the epidural process without recourse to injection of contrast medium by the upper route (Fig. 20).

The diffusion of neoplastic cells in the C.S.F., most often due to a breaking into the leptomeninx or the ventricular walls at the cerebral level, can lead to arachnoiditic lesions (Fig. 21) characterized by irregularities in the caliber and by conglomerates of the nerve roots of the cauda equina, these being generally involved by the metastatic process, as is the spinal cord. This kind of lesion, frequently encountered in cases of metastatic diffusion of primary tumors of the CNS, is also encountered in metastases from extraneural tumors. Differential diagnosis from chronic arachnoiditis can be difficult. The absence of atrophy, or even increased size, of the visible roots suggests neoplastic infiltration (Fig. 21).

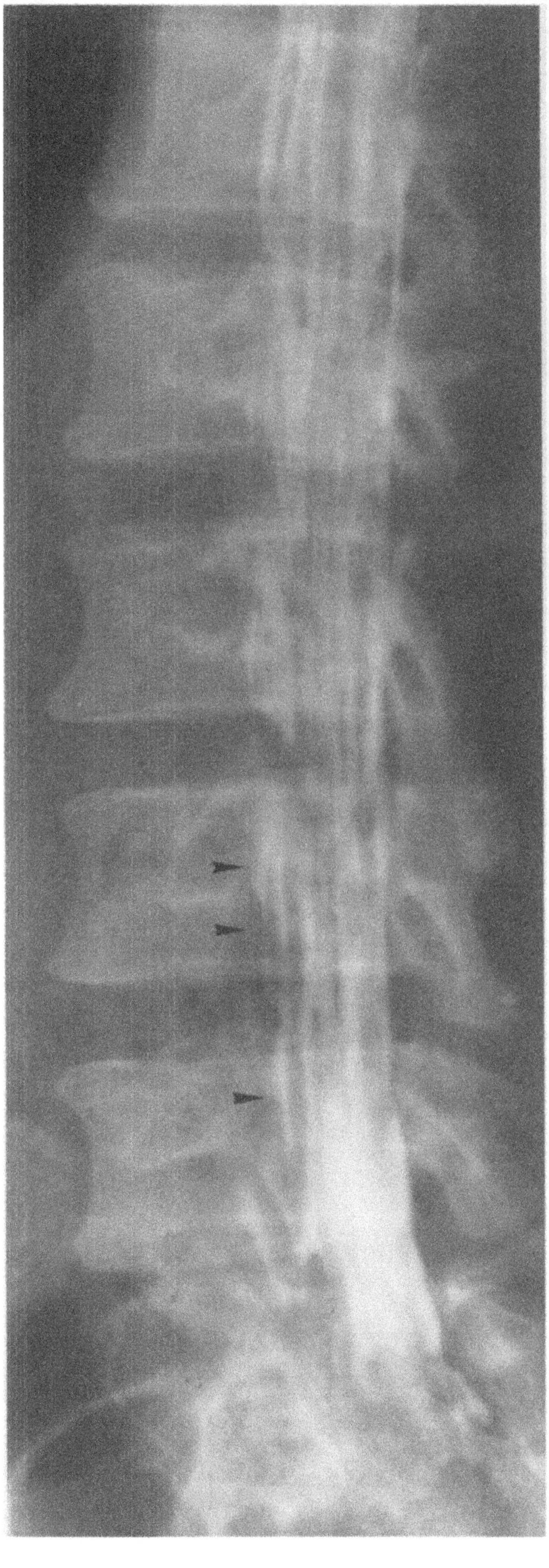

a

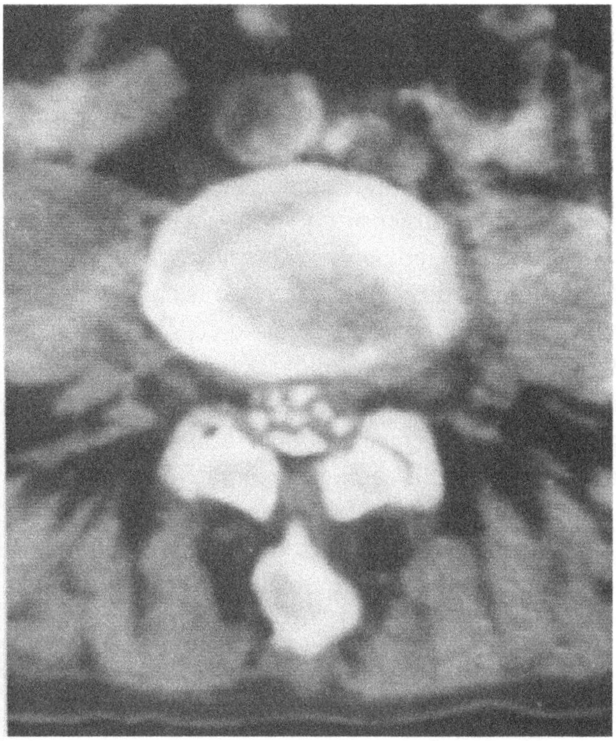

b

Fig. 21a, b. Leptomeningeal metastatic dissemination of a synoviosarcoma. Myelography (**a**) shows a conglomerate image of the roots of the cauda equina with thickened appearance (*arrows*). CT after myelography (**b**) shows the "inverted" image typical for arachnoiditis: presence of some isolated dense areas of contrast medium at the center of the roots conglomerate

E. Differential Diagnosis

The differential diagnosis of metastatic lesions of the spine must take account of primary tumors, inflammatory lesions, and certain degenerative changes.

There is no absolute radiological criterion for metastatic lesions, especially in isolation, either with standard radiology or with CT. The lytic lesions must also be differentiated from primitive tumoral conditions and from infectious lesions; these can also lead to epidural infiltrations. The condensing lesions must also be differentiated from primary tumors, generally benign, and also from the sometimes misleading degenerative changes.

In numerous cases a careful anamnesis, comparison of old and recent radiographs, and the juxtaposition of different techniques of investigation could resolve the problem.

Primary tumors are discussed elsewhere (STIENON and JEANMART, this volume).

I. Infectious Lesions

The vertebral column is one of the most frequent sites of osteomyelitis (staphyloccocal, caused by less common bacteria, of tuberculous). The lesions, often initially destructive, can subsequently be accompanied by condensation (Fig. 22). One of their characteristics that is useful in differential diagnosis is the frequency of disk involvement (spondylodiscitis). Once affected, the disk space can totally disappear in subsequent stages, giving the appearance of "fusion" of the two involved adjacent vertebral bodies (Fig. 23a).

Metastatic lesions, in contrast, usually spare the intervertebral disk. The infectious lesions can also give rise to images of paravertebral "spindles" owing to spread to the adjacent soft tissues. Voluminous paravertebral masses, sometimes calcified, similar to abcesses may thus be encountered, particularly in tuberculous spondylodiscitis. Deformation of the affected vertebra is frequent and can give way to major alterations of statics (Fig. 23a). Epidural infiltration is not exceptional in these infectious lesions, spreading fairly often directly to the canal from the adjacent spondylodiscitis lesions, but sometimes from some distance away by a metastatic dissemination mechanism (Fig. 23c).

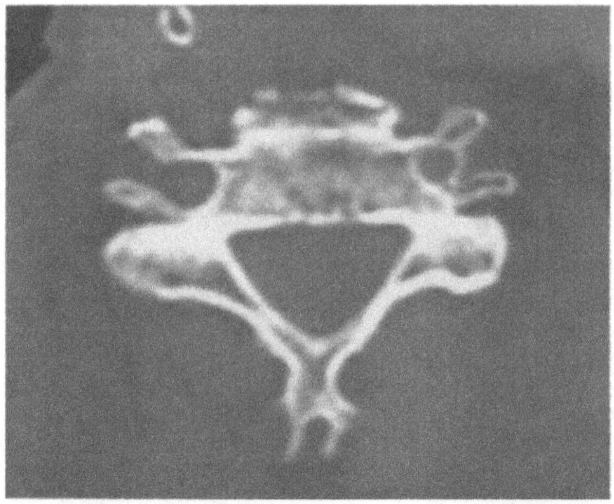
a

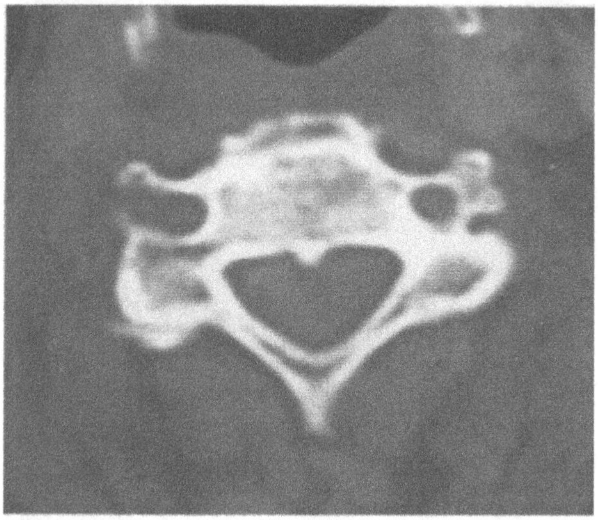
b

Fig. 22a, b. Subacute osteomyelitis in a patient presenting with intense cervical pain and a septic condition. He had undergone surgery several years before for thyroid cancer. Blood cultures revealed septicemia with *Staphylococcus aureus*. Isotopic studies with labeled white cells showed fixation in the upper cervical region. There was no evidence of any osseous metastases on radiologic examination of the skeleton.
a CT at this time showed no destructive or densifying lesion at C4; **b** 42 days after the onset of antibiotic therapy high-resolution CT control demonstrates irregular, confluent areas of bone densification in the vertebral body of C4. With treatment, pain had almost totally disappeared, but a control scintiscan with labeled white cells remained positive.
No definitive diagnosis was available because no puncture was done, but clinical and radiologic courses strongly suggest subacute osteomyelitis

II. Degenerative Lesions

The problem of confusion between isolated degenerative lesions and osseous metastatic lesions of the vertebral column rarely arises. In the majority of

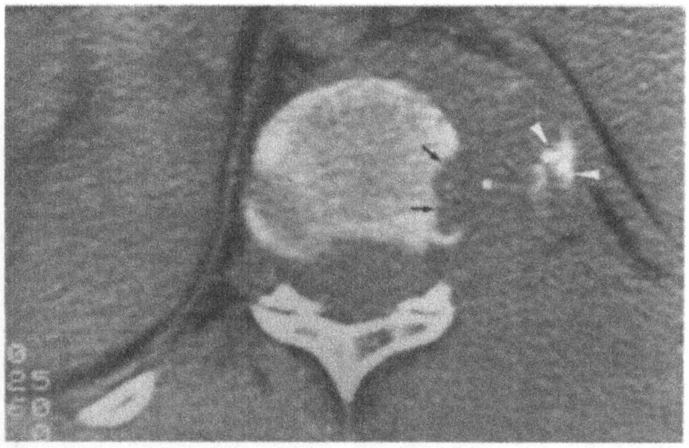
b

Fig. 23a–c. Pott's disease and distant tuberculous epiduritis. This 25-year-old man was admitted with progressive-onset tetraparesis. Conventional x-ray of the spine (**a**) on admission shows a marked destructive lesion of T10 and T11 with asymmetrical collapse of the vertebral bodies and densifying changes, also seen in T9. Note the total absence of the intervertebral disk space at T10–T11 level. There was a large extension of the tuberculous abscess in the paravertebral soft tissues (essentially on the right) with calcifications (*arrowheads*). CT clearly demonstrates this soft tissue condensation. **b** At T12 calcifications already seen on standard radiographs are visible (*arrowheads*) and there is marginal effraction of the vertebral body (*arrows*).
c In the same patient cervical myelography was performed, detecting a complete myelographic block, seemingly of epidural origin, at C3 (*arrows*). Surgery later confirmed an epidural tuberculous granuloma, displacing the medulla backward and compressing it. The patient made a complete recovery

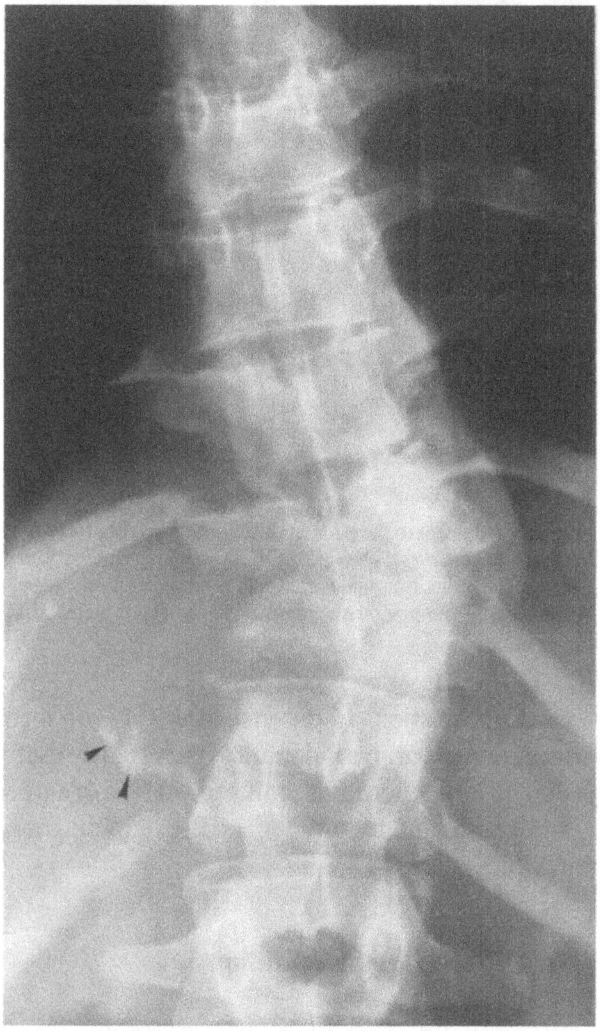
a

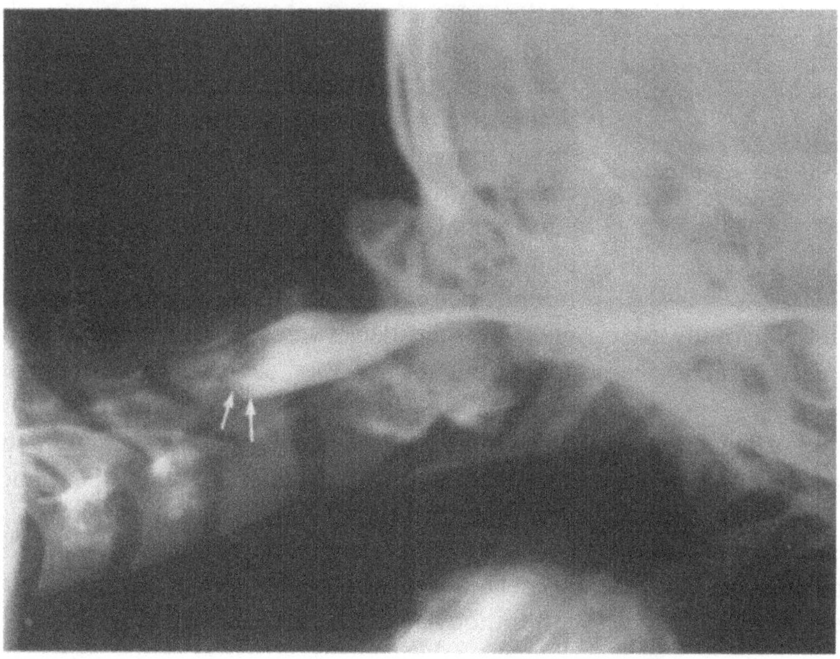
c

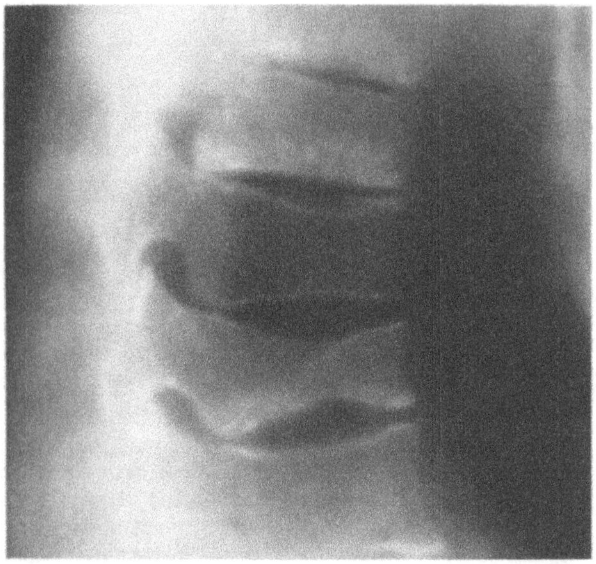

a

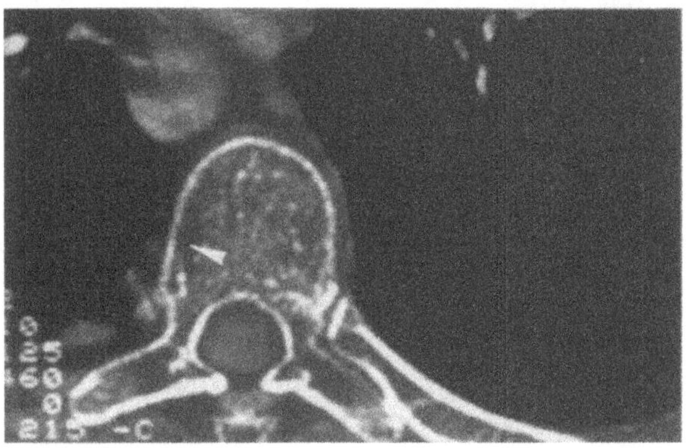

b

Fig. 24a, b. Extensive osteoporosis in a 40-year-old known male alcoholic with very poor general condition, presenting with severe back pain in the thoracic section. **a** Standard x-rays show extensive lesions of osteoporosis, with collapse of numerous vertebrae. **b** CT shows very regular rarefaction of the bone texture without any cortical disruption or replacement by solid tumor tissue. There are, however, some areas of fatty replacement, with typical lipidic densities (negative values on Hounsfield scale: *arrowhead*).
Comparison with Fig. 18a shows that differential diagnosis by voncentional x-rays is very difficult in the presence of diffuse infiltration (e.g., by myeloma). In such situations CT seems to be essential for confirmation of a benign etiology

cases, the careful observation of radiographs, perhaps compared with computerized tomographs, allows the right diagnosis.

On the other hand, the presence of degenerative changes can lead to particular difficulty in the detection of small adjacent metastatic lesions. Densifying changes in shape caused by degeneration adjacent to the vertebral end plate can hide the small lytic lesions or be confused with a localized

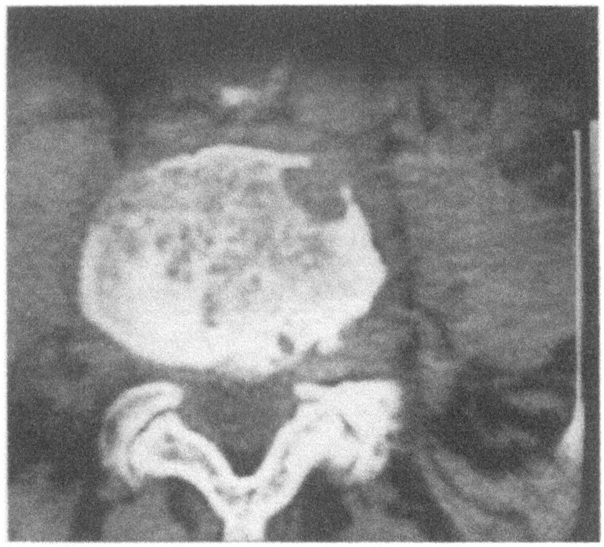

Fig. 25. Adjacent to the plate of this lumbar vertebra (with well-defined degeneratice changes), CT shows a marginal lytic area with cortical disruption and contiguous paravertebral fusion of tumor tissue (homogeneous, density 30–40 HU); metastasis

blastic infiltration. In the first case, CT with high-resolution programs is doubtless particularly useful (Fig. 25). In other cases, only the analysis of earlier radiographs and followup make the right diagnosis possible.

III. Diffuse Demineralization

Differential diagnosis between diffuse demineralization of the vertebral column (most often of osteoporotic origin) and diffuse neoplastic infiltrations or supplementary focal infiltrations is sometimes extremely difficult. Collapse of osteoporotic origin is frequent and does not present specific characteristics. Conventional CT, in view of its poor spatial and densitic resolution, is often disappointing. High-resolution CT, if it shows regular rarefaction of the mineral stroma with no replacement by solid densities but with replacement by zones of lipidic densities, could suggest osteoporosis (Fig. 24). However, the CT aspect of diffused infiltrations on the microscopic scale should be confirmed by further studies. On the other hand, when the CT examination reveals localized replacement of the stroma by solid tissue and the existence of a cortical disruption, the neoplastic infiltration can easily be confirmed (Fig. 25).

References

1. Abrams HL (1957) The vertebral and azygos venous systems, and some variations in systemic venous return. Radiology 69:508–526
2. Anderson RK (1951) Diodrast studies of the vertebral and cranial venous system to show their probable role in spread of metastases. J Neurosurg 8:411–422
3. Arseni CN, Simionescu MD, Horwath L (1959) Tumors of the spine. A follow-up study of 350 patients with neurosurgical considerations. Acta Psychiatr Neurol Scand 34:398–410
4. Barron KD, Hirano A, Araki S, Terry RD (1959) Experiences with metastatic neoplasms involving the spinal cord. Neurology 9:91–106
5. Batson OV (1940) Function of vertebral veins and their role in spread of metastases. Ann Surg 112:138–149
6. Batson OV (1942) The role of the vertebral veins in metastatic processes. Ann Intern Med 16:38–45
7. Batson OV (1941) The vertebral vein system as a mechanism for the spread of metastases. Am J Roentgenol 48:715–718
8. Chade HO (1976) Metastatic tumors of the spine and spinal cord. In: Vinken PJ, Bruyn GW (eds) Handbook of clinical neurology, vol 20. North-Holland, Amsterdam, pp 415–433
9. Chandler HC, French LA, Peyton WT (1954) Surgical treatment of metastatic tumors of the spine. Ann Surg 140:197–199
10. Coman DR, De Long RP (1951) Role of the vertebral venous system in metastasis of cancer to spinal column; experiments with tumor-cells suspensions in rats and rabbits Cancer 4:610–618
11. Copeland MM, Geschickter OF (1963) Malignant bone tumors: primary and metastatic CA 13 149:187–232
12. De Wilde A, Frühling J, Osteaux M, Jeanmart L, Henry J (1976) Confrontations de résultats de la scintigraphie osseuse et de la radiographie systématique du squelette dans la recherche des métastases au cours de l'evolution des néoplasies mammaires. J Belge Radiol 59/2:131–138
13. Deemarsky LY, Chernomordikova MF (1971) Clinical and Roentgenologic picture of the alterations obtained in the treatment of breast cancer osseous metastases. Cancer 28:282
14. Drury RAB, Palmer PH, Highman WJ (1964) Carcinomatous metastasis to the vertebral bodies. J Clin Pathol 17:448–457
15. Epstein BS (1974) The vertebral column. In: Hodes PJ (ed) An atlas of tumor radiology. Hodes PJ (ed) Year Book Medical Publishers, Chicago
16. Fornasier VL, Horne JG (1975) Metastatis to the vertebral column. Cancer 36:590
17. Gilbert H, Apuzzo M, Marshall L (1978) Neoplastic epidural spinal cord compression. A current perspective. Jama 240:2771–2773
18. Gordan GS, Fitzpatrick ME, Lubick WP (1967) Identification of osteolytic sterols in human breast cancer. Trans Assoc Am Physicians 80:183
19. Guyer PB, Westbury H (1968) The myelographic appearance of spinal cord metastases. Br J Radiol 41:615–619
20. Helms CA, Cann CE, Brunelle FO, Gilula LA, Chafetz N, Genant HK (1981) Detection of bone-marrow metastases using quantitative computed tomography. Radiology 140:745–750
21. Jacobson HG, Poppel MH, Shapiro JH, Grossberger S (1958) The vertebral pedicle sign: a roentgen finding to differenciate metastatic carcinoma from multiple myeloma. AmJ 80:817–821
22. Jaffe HJ (1958) Tumors and tumorous conditions of the bones and joints. Lea and Febiger, Philadelphia, p 589
23. Loer F, Graf Steinbock-Femor N (1980) Der Stellenwert der Computertomographie bei der Diagnostik von Skelettmetastasen. Dtsch Med Wochenschr 26/27:937–938
24. Longeval E, Hildebrand J, Vollont GH (1975) Early diagnosis of metastases in the epidural space. Acta Neurochir (Wien) 31:177–184
25. Matelart AL, Osteaux M, De Wilde A (1979) Unusual and early aspects of bone metastasis. J Belge Radiol 62:35–40
26. Milch RA, Changus GW (1956) Response to tumor invasion. Cancer 9:340
27. Mullins G, Flynn JPG, El-Mahdi AM, McQueen JD, Owens AH (1971) Malignant lymphoma of the spinal epidural space. Ann Intern Med 74:416–423
28. Odelberg-Johnson O (1959) Osteosclerotic changes in myelomatosis: report of a case. Acta Radiol (Stockh) 52:139–144
29. Onofrio BM, Svien HJ (1976) Solitary and multiple vertebral myelomas. In: Vinken PJ, Bruyn GW (eds) Handbook of Clinical Neurology, vol 20. North-Holland, Amsterdam pp 9–18
30. Prentice WB, Kiefer SA, Gold LHA, Bjornson RGB (1973) Myelographic characteristics of metastasis to the spinal cord and cauda equina. AJR 118:682–689
31. Rogers L, Heard G (1958) Intrathecal spinal metastases (rare tumors) Br J Surg 45:317–320
32. Sellwood RB (1971) The radiological approach to metastatic cancer of the brain and spine. Br J Radiol 45:647–651
33. Stoll B, Parboo S (1983) Bone metastasis: monitoring and treatment. Raven, New York
34. Swanson DA, Bernardino ME (1982) "Silent" osseous metastases in renal cell carcinoma: value of computerized tomography. Urology 20/2:208–212
35. Takakura K, Keiji S, Shuntaro H, Asao H (1932) Metastatic tumors of the spinal canal. In: Metastatic tumors of the central nervous system. Igaku-Shoin, Tokyo, pp 280–295
36. Takakura K, Keiji S, Shuntard H, Asao H (1982) Metastatic tumors in the vertebral canal (pathology). In: Metastatic tumors of the central nervous system. Igaku-Shoin, Tokyo, pp 93–101
37. Torma T (1957) Malignant tumors of the spine and spinal extradural space. A study based on 250 histologically verified cases. Acta Chir Scand [Suppl] 225:1–138
38. Ushio Y, Posner R, Posner JB, Shapiro WR (1977) Experimental spinal cord compression by epidural neoplasms. Neurology 27:422–429
39. Verity GL (1968) Neurologic manifestations and complications of lymphoma. Radiol Clin North Am 6:672–676
40. Waldenström J (1970) Diagnosis and treatment of multiple myeloma. Grune and Stratton, New York
41. Willis RA (1973) The spread of tumors in the human body. Butterworth, London
42. Wilner D (1982) Metastatic tumors in the skeleton; cancer metastasis to bone. In: Radiology of bone tumors and allied disorders. Saunders, Philadelphia, pp 3642–3882
43. Wilner D (1982) (ed) Malignant hematologic and lymphoid disorders of bone. In: Radiology of bone tumors and allied disorders. Saunders, Philadelphia pp 2859–2940

Metastatic Disease of the Spine: The Contribution of Bone Scintigraphy

J. FRÜHLING

A. Introduction

The skeleton is one of the most frequent sites of tumor metastasis, only the lung and the liver being more frequently affected.

The most important pathologic and diagnostic aspects of metastatic bone disease have been treated recently in the book *Bone Metastasis* edited by WEISS and GILBERT, [32], and according to several collections of data discussed in this work the metastatic process is characterized as a complex event involving cell release from the primary tumor; dissemination of these cells by blood or lymphatic current; implantation and survival of the tumor cells in the new environment; and their development into a secondary tumor mass. Metastases have a predilection for certain sites within the skeleton; neoplastic deposits are particularly frequent in the axial skeleton, and especially in the spine. This is dependent on several factors, which are discussed in detail in other chapters of the present work. Nevertheless, we stress here the importance of the vertebral venous system, which has been (re)discovered and described by BATSON [4]. This pathway constitutes a preferential route for the transmission of released tumor cells and thus explains the high incidence of metastatic disease in the spine and the spinal canal.

Among the diagnostic methods devoted to in vivo detection of bone metastases, the recent increase in the use of scintigraphy, or radionuclide bone imaging (RBI) is attributable to significant technologic improvements in the field of tracers and imaging equipment, leading to a more valuable contribution of bone scintigraphy owing to its ability to detect metastatic bone disease earlier than other medical imaging technique can [3, 8, 25].

The aim of the present chapter is to summarize the results obtained with RBI in the detection of bone metastases affecting the spine, based on the most important papers available in the literature, with special reference to the differences in the three main segments (cervical, thoracic, lumbar) of the vertebral column. Futhermore, we shall discuss our own results on the same topic, based on about 2500 verified bone scintigrams concerned with the most frequent at least in our institute — sites of neoplastic conditions: breast, lung, head and neck, gastrointestinal, prostate, and thyroid cancers, lymphomas, and melanomas. Finally, some technical aspects of RBI will also be considered to complete the information for the interested reader with no specific training as nuclear medicine specialist.

B. Materials and Methods

I. General Considerations

As bone seeking tracers, ^{85}Sr-, ^{87m}Sr-, ^{18}F-, ^{67}Ga-, and ^{99m}Tc-labeled phosphates and phosphonates have been in large-scale clinical use since the introduction of RBI into current medical practice in the late 1960s. In fact, ^{99m}Tc-labeled agents can be considered as the products of choice, especially for the following reasons: the monoenergetic emission (140 KeV) of ^{99m}Tc is well suited to the currently used imaging device (Anger-type camera); ^{99m}Tc has a short half-life (6 h), and emits no beta rays, so that the radiation dose to the patients is low; the blood clearance of these molecules is fast enough and the target nontarget ratio is advantageous. Among the various ^{99m}Tc-labeled compounds the pyrophosphate molecule was used at first with large success; at present the products in most frequent use are the various diphosphonates. Clinically useful and diagnostically helpful studies can be carried out with doses varying between 15 and 20 mCi (555–740 MBq) ^{99m}Tc-labeled products, according to the number of examinations to be performed, to the age and clinical condition of the patients, to the pathology encountered, and to the valid legal regulations in the different countries.

The imaging device can be a rectilinear scanner, an Anger-type γ-camera, or a SPECT-type tomocamera. In general hospital practice bone scintigraphy involves anterior and posterior total-body images obtained with a scanning γ-camera in the majority of cases, complemented if appropriate by selected "spot" images of regions of particular interest. The quantitative evaluation of the data collected is possible, since most nuclear medicine departments have access to a medical computer, but the clinical diagnosis is generally established on the basis of the analogous images. Metabolic investigations [1, 10, 11, 27] are not yet sufficiently widely used in the area of metastasis detection to be considered a clinical routine.

II. Specific Data

1. Patients Studied

In all 2532 patients entered into this study. All have had a histologically proven neoplastic disease, the sample including: 752 cases of breast carcinoma, 656 lung carcinomas, 295 melanomas, 257 head and neck cancers, 210 cancers of the digestive tract, 204 lymphomas, 85 prostatic, and 73 thyroid cancers. Most patients had undergone several scintigraphic examinations (up to 19). Their condition was classified as metastatic or not, according to the last verified bone scintigraphy. Scintigraphy was verified by x-ray examination (conventional or tomographic), x-ray CT scan, biopsy, surgery, or autopsy performed during the same observation period (± 6 weeks) as the last bone scintigram. In some cases positive neurologic findings concordant with active bone lesions localized by the nuclear bone study, or lesions which appeared on roentgenograms several months later but had been predicted by the scintigraphic "hot spots" were also accepted as verification.

2. Scintigraphic Technique

^{87m}Sr was used as tracer between 1970 and 1974, when the dose injected was 1–4 mCi (37–148 MBq); this applied to 53 cases, or 2.1% of the whole population studied. A further 228 patients (= 9.0%) were studied by means of ^{99m}Tc-pyrophosphate during the period 1974–1976. Since 1976 we have used ^{99m}Tc-methylendiphosphonate (MDP), this population constituting 88.9% of all cases examined. The dose of the ^{99m}Tc-labeled phosphates injected varies between 14 and 22 mCi (= 518–814 MBq). About 33% of all patients were examined with a standard γ-camera [25 cm useful diameter, 19 photomultipliers (PMs)] giving 12–15 spot images, omitting arms, knees, tibias, and feet. In the other 1688 patients, studied by a large-field (40 cm head diameter, 37 PMs) moving γ-camera, a posterior whole-body image and anterior static views of skull, thorax, pelvis, and femora were recorded. The delay between injection and scintiscanning varied between 2 ½ and 6 h.

The evaluation was based on optical examination of the analogous records (x-ray films or Polaroid-type photographs) completed by quantitative uptake measurements taken in selected areas in less than 5% of all cases. In these last patients a 30% higher fixation level than in normal bone was considered significantly pathologic. Scintigraphic findings were recorded without knowledge of the x-ray examination results.

C. Results and Comments

I. Data from the Literature

Table 1 presents the incidence of metastatic bone disease localized in the spine or in its main segments, according to nonscintigraphic methods and the authors most frequently cited in the literature [2, 6, 16, 17, 19, 28, 30, 34]. When these results are considered it must be taken into account that the number of these papers is relatively small; they are based (except for two) on limited patient series; and since autopsy is being the verification method generally used they are concerned with terminal cases. Thus, the results cited correspond to a higher metastatic incidence than is seen in daily clinical practice, where patients are examined before, or in

Table 1. Incidence of bone metastases in various neoplastic diseases, established by autopsy or x-ray examination

Author [Reference]	Tumor	Verification method	Number of cases	Total spinal involvement	Cervical vertebrae	Thoracic vertebrae	Lumbar vertebrae
Kaufmann, 1902 [17]	Prostate cancer	Autopsy	34	–	–	56%	79%
Simpson, 1926 [30]	Thyroid cancer	Autopsy	77	32%	–	–	–
Pürckhauer 1929 [28]	Prostate cancer	Autopsy	30	90%	–	–	–
Aufses 1930 [2]	Rectal cancer	Autopsy	24	33%	–	–	–
Lenz and Freid 1931 [19]	Breast cancer	Autopsy and x-ray	81	59%	–	–	–
Drury et al. 1964 [6]	Miscellaneous	Autopsy	575	33%	–	–	–
Holmes and Fouts 1970 [16]	Primary site unknown	Autopsy	686	5.1%	–	–	–
Willis 1973 [34]	Miscellaneous	Autopsy	68	62%	22%	36%	53%

the initial phase of metastatic disease or during treatment.

The figures confirm the high incidence of metastasis to bone in breast and prostate carcinoma, but there is a clear difference (1:2) between the two main groups with miscellaneous tumors. The rare segmental analyses revealed an increasing tendency to metastatic involvement from the higher to the lower vertebrae. It should be underlined, for interest, that the general incidence of spinal metastatic disease in the papers cited (except in one article) varies in multiples of 30%. This same tendency (an anecdotal one?) persists in Table 2, which summarizes the incidence of bone metastases determined in the spine and in its three main segments by means of bone scintigraphy, an in vivo investigation technique. Table 2 contains most of the relevant data in the literature on this topic, and also reflects the evolution of nuclear medicine during the last 10 years; nevertheless, it allows the following statements.

The number of cases studied is sufficient, but only breast carcinomas and lymphomas are well represented; according to our knowledge, for head and neck cancers, gastrointestinal carcinomas, and prostate and lung carcinomas no detailed segmental studies of metastatic involvement were available. As far as the segmental involvement is concerned the highest figures are found in Galasko's work [13], which seems logical since, the clinical population was made up exclusively of patients with advanced breast carcinoma and the tracer used was the most favorable one (^{18}F).

In early breast cancer the corresponding figures

Table 2. Incidence of bone metastases in the spine and in its three main segments as established by bone scintigraphy (Data collected from the literature)

Author [Reference]	Tumor	Verification method	Scintigraphic product	Number of cases	Total spinal involvement	Cervical vertebrae	Thoracic vertebrae	Lumbar vertebrae
Galasko 1972 [13]	Advanced breast carcinoma	Scintigraphy and x-ray	^{18}F	127	–	26%	72%	68%
Wiebe and Erbe 1973 [33]	Thyroid carcinoma	Scintigraphy and x-ray	^{131}I	34	32%	–	–	–
Rampon et al. 1974 [29]	Miscellaneous	Scintigraphy and x-ray	^{99m}TC-PP	101	–	2%	24%	29%
Eggenstein et al. 1978 [7]	Hodkin's lymphoma	Scintigraphy	^{99m}TC-PP	67	2 out of 14 SC +	–	–	–
	Non-Hodking's lymphoma			64	1 out of 12 SC +	–	–	–
Liedholm et al. 1978 [20]	Early breast carcinoma	Scintigraphy	^{99m}TC-PP and DP	467	–	4.5%	9.4%	9.0%
Nomura et al. 1978 [24]	Breast carcinoma	Scintigraphy	^{99m}TC-PP	224	–	4%	12%	19%
Wahner et al 1980 [31]	Myeloma	Scintigraphy and x-ray	^{99m}TC-EHDP	27	–	30%	48%	37%
Fon et al. 1981 [12]	Melanoma	Scintigraphy and x-ray	^{99m}TC-DP	145	–	1.4%	10.3%	5.5%
Wilson and Calhoun 1981 [35]	Miscellaneous	Scintigraphy	^{99m}TC-PP	318	65%	–	–	–
Newcomer et al. 1982 [23]	Hodkin's lymphoma	Scintigraphy, x-ray, biopsy	Non-ment.	118	–	1.7%	12.7%	5.9%

are clearly lower [20, 24], but the proportions in the different vertebral segments remain relatively constant. As far as the segmental distribution is concerned, the cervical spine presents the lowest degree of metastatic involvement everywhere, the absolute figures being below 5% for each cancer studied except advanced breast carcinoma and myeloma. The thoracic and lumbar segments have quite a similar tendency to bone metastases; thoracic involvement is clearly more frequent with melanomas [12] and HK lymphomas [23], whereas according to Nomura [24], in his patients with breast carcinoma the lumbar spine is the site of significantly more metastases. All these data seem to confirm the increasing "vertebral metastatic gradient" from the skull to the sacrum, especially when this is expressed in other ways than as percentage of metastases/segment, e. g., as percentage of metastases/vertebra. According to this last calculation the metastatic involvement of cervical vertebrae will be nearer to that of the thoracic spine, whereas lumbar vertebrae will show the highest incidence.

II. Personal Results

Our own results following analysis of more than 8000 bone scintigrams recorded between 1970 and 1983 in 2532 patients, among them 1036 (= 40.9 %) with proven bone metastases, are summarized by Figs. 1 and 2 and illustrated by Figs. 3–8.

Figure 1 shows histograms giving the absolute number of cases of bone metastases, their localizations (spinal or not), their correlation to other osseous localizations (metastases elsewhere combined with vertebral involvement or metastases in the spine only), and finally the proportions of isolated versus multiple spinal metastases, as a function of the neoplastic disease studied. These data allow the following statements.

The entire population can be subdivided into three main groups if the number of patients with each cancer studied is considered: two large patient subgroups (breast and lung carcinoma); four medium-sized subgroups (200–300 cases: melanoma, head and neck carcinoma, gastrointestinal carcinoma, and lymphomas); and finally, two groups with less than 100 cases each (prostate and thyroid carcinoma).

With respect to the general incidence of metastatic bone disease, two cancers show a high value: prostatic carcinoma (nearly 73 %) and breast carcinoma (around 47 %). All six other groups have a surprisingly similar incidence, metastatic involvement of bones varying between 30.1 % and 38.9 %.

From the aspect of anatomic distribution of metastases (with or without spinal component), three main groups can be distinguished: in head and neck cancers, lymphomas, and melanomas 46 %–47 % of the patients had bone metastases without any vertebral localization. From this point of view, the two cancers with the highest absolute incidence of bone metastasis (breast and prostate) also have the smallest numbers of localizations (11.4 % and 19.2 %) without spinal involvement, whereas lung, thyroid, and digestive tract cancers exhibit an intermediate position with 25 %–34 % of bone metastases localized exclusively outside the vertebral column.

When there is spinal involvement two main types of patients can be differentiated: cases with metastases localized in the spine only (regardless of whether there are one or more pathologic vertebrae) and those where the bone metastases are located both in the spine and elsewhere in the skeleton. In proportion to the whole population, in all kinds of cancers the incidence of patients with metastases in the vertebral column only is low (2.8 %–5.3 %), except for the group with lung carcinoma, where the proportion is over 10 %; the 9.1 % in the thyroid cancer group has no statistical significance, referring to 2 cases only. In the majority of patients (5 of the 8 cancers studied) the existence of spinal metastases is combined with other localizations elsewhere, this kind of multiple localization representing 59.1 %–75.5 % of cases. Three cancers (lymphomas, melanomas, head and neck carcinoma), constitute a specific unit with lower and quite similar incidences (48 %–50 %) of miscellaneous (spinal and elsewhere) metastatic bone disease, and these also exhibit a relatively high percentage of metastases without spinal components (see above).

Consideration of the number of vertebrae affected with no reference to whether or not they are combined with extraspinal involvement reveals that most patients have several vertebrae affected by metastases, especially when the primary tumor is in the prostate, breast or lung. These three cancers also have the highest absolute incidence of bone metastasis. Head and neck cancers, melanomas, thyroid carcinomas, and lymphomas occur in more cases with isolated vertebral localizations; three of these four cancers are also characterized by a lower degree of vertebral involvement, as stated above. Thus, in a given cancer, the lower the incidence of spinal involvement the more often isolated vertebral localizations are encountered.

The second figure represents the anatomic distribution of the metastatic bone lesions by the three main vertebral segments, as established by bone scintigraphy in the eight different neoplastic dis-

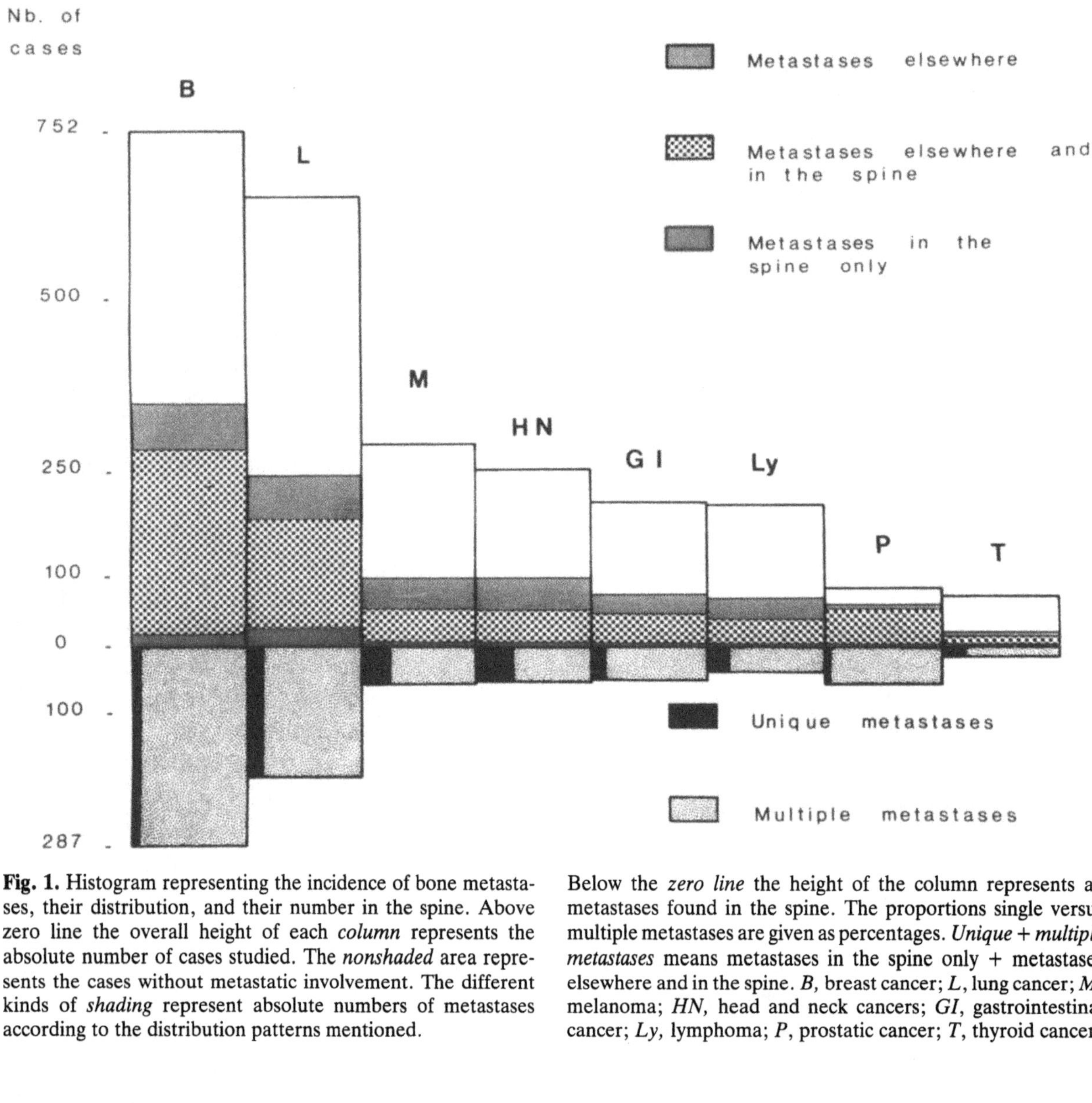

Fig. 1. Histogram representing the incidence of bone metastases, their distribution, and their number in the spine. Above zero line the overall height of each *column* represents the absolute number of cases studied. The *nonshaded* area represents the cases without metastatic involvement. The different kinds of *shading* represent absolute numbers of metastases according to the distribution patterns mentioned. Below the *zero line* the height of the column represents all metastases found in the spine. The proportions single versus multiple metastases are given as percentages. *Unique + multiple metastases* means metastases in the spine only + metastases elsewhere and in the spine. *B*, breast cancer; *L*, lung cancer; *M*, melanoma; *HN*, head and neck cancers; *GI*, gastrointestinal cancer; *Ly*, lymphoma; *P*, prostatic cancer; *T*, thyroid cancer

eases studied, with the corresponding main values computed from all cases presenting the same type of neoplastic vertebral bone involvement (unique or multiple). The distribution of 89 localizations was studied in the group "Unique metastases", whereas the results in the section "multiple metastases" derive from the analysis of more than 1800 pathologic vertebral localizations (identified in 651 patients, one block of several involved adjacent vertebrae being considered one localization).

In the category "unique metastases" the cervical segment shows the lowest metastatic incidence, the individual figures corresponding to the different cancerous diseases being insignificant in view of the low absolute number of cervical vertebrae affected. The thoracic and lumbar involvement is equal as demonstrated by the average value, but the variations among the cancers studied are quite substantial (0–85.7%) in the thoracic segment and 14.3–83.3% in the lumbar segment) for the same reason as in the cervical segment.

In the case of multiple metastases the incidence of cervical involvement is higher in proportion (16.4%), whereas the incidence of thoracic vertebral bone metastases is 10% higher than in the lumbar segment. Thanks to the relatively high number of metastatic localizations encountered,

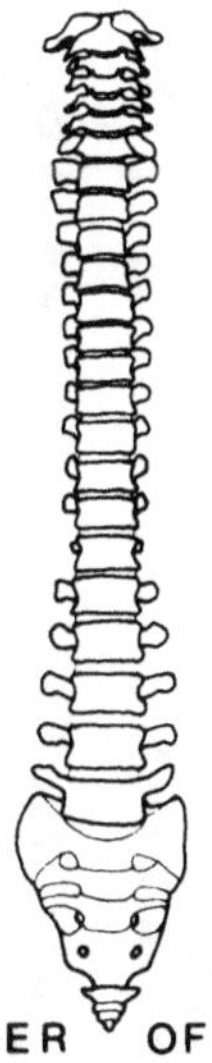

	UNIQUE METASTASES									MULTIPLE METASTASES								
Av	T	P	Ly	GI	HN	M	L	B		B	L	M	HN	GI	Ly	P	T	Av
11,2	0	0	0	16,7	11,8	15,4	13	11,2	C	13	12,1	26,2	16,7	14,3	18,5	27,6	17,4	16,4
42,7	33,3	50	85,7	0	35,3	23,1	43,5	61,1	Th	48,2	52,8	36,9	42,6	44,2	44,5	37,9	47,8	46,1
46,1	66,7	50	14,3	83,3	52,9	61,5	43,5	27,7	Lb	38,8	35,1	36,9	40,7	41,5	37	34,7	34,8	37,5
NUMBER OF CASES	3	2	7	6	17	13	23	18		269	165	41	36	44	31	53	12	

Fig. 2. Segmental distribution of spinal bone metastases expressed as percentages of total number of cases studied in a given cancer with vertebral metastatic disease and according to the type of metastatic involvement (single or multiple). *C*, cervical; *Th*, thoracic; *Lb*, lumbar vertebrae. *B*, breast cancer; *L*, lung cancer; *M*, melanoma; *HN*, head and neck cancer; *GI*, gastrointestinal cancer; *Ly*, lymphoma; *P*, prostatic cancer; *T*, thyroid cancer. *Av*, mean value in a given segment, expressed as a percentage of all cases presenting the same type of neoplastic vertebral bone involvement (single or multiple)

the distribution can be analyzed in the individual groups according to the basic neoplastic disease. Thus, in the cervical segment, melanomas and prostatic carcinoma have the highest incidence, the extreme values reaching from the simple more than to the double. The melanomas and prostatic cancers metastasized to the thoracic spine in less than 40% of cases, whereas lung cancer patients had the highest (52.8%) incidence of thoracic localizations. The incidence of metastatic disease in the lumbar vertebrae (average 37.5%) is remarkably stable, not varying by more than 4% either way in all eight diseases studied.

When all metastatic localizations (single and multiple) were combined (1282 foci with segmental distribution), the overall distribution was found to be the following: 16.07% of all metastases were localized in the cervical spine; 45.87%, in the thoracic segment; and 38.06% in the lumbar vertebrae. The incidence calculated as the percentage of metastases per single vertebra in each part of the spine gives the clearest expression of the susceptibility of each individual segment to metastatic disease. This incidence is 2.29% in the cervical segment, 3.82% in the thoracic segment, and finally 7.61% in the lumbar section. These figures confirm the downward gradient quite regularly found, which seems to be characteristic of metastatic disease in the vertebral column and which was also seen when the results displayed in Table 2 were analyzed.

D. Discussion

RBI is now established as one of the most important diagnostic procedures in detecting active pathologic processes of the skeleton. The suspicion of malignant disease is the main indication for bone imaging in most cases [9].

The essential role of RBI is due to its high sensitivity, which derives from the use of true physiologic markers of bone metabolism [22, 26].

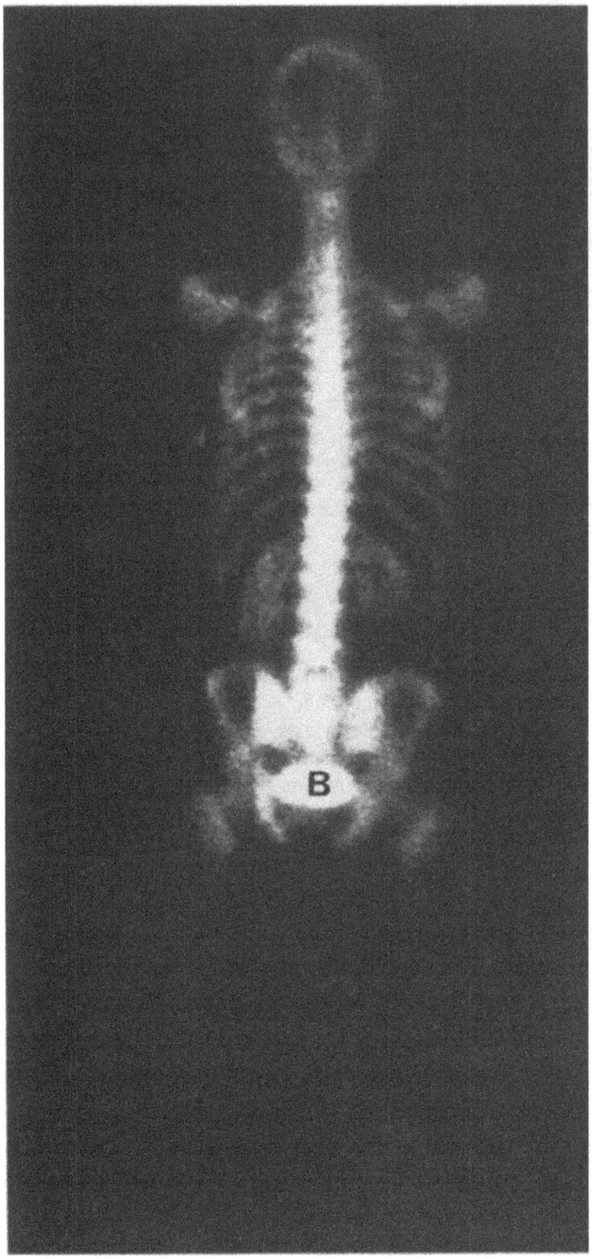

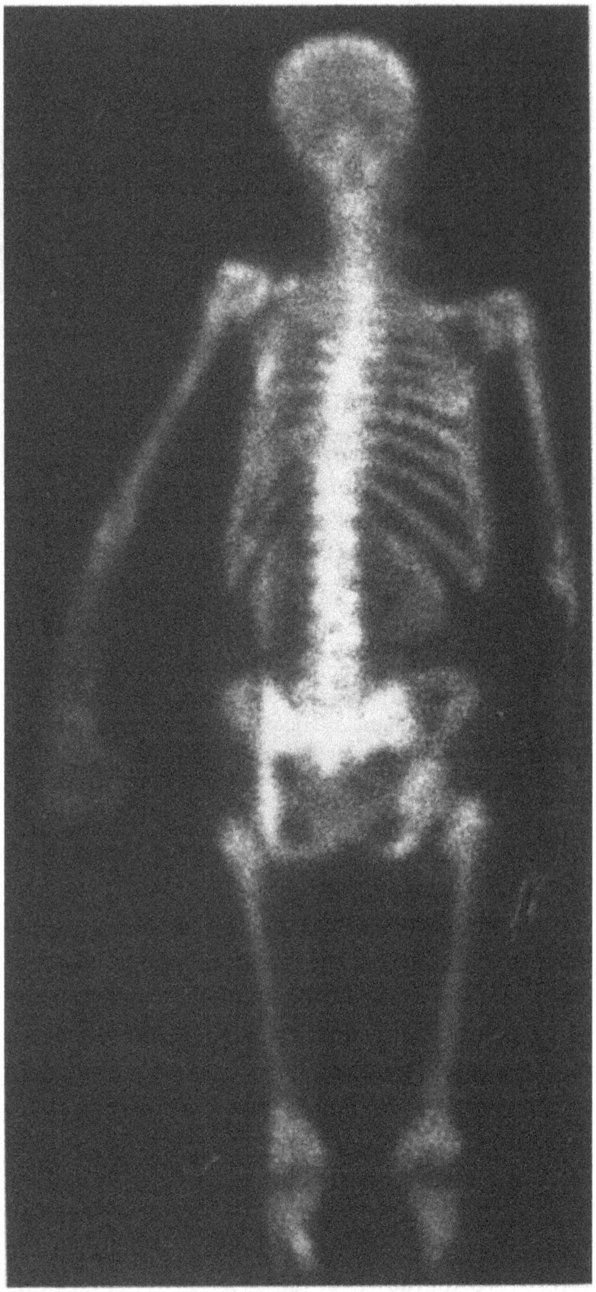

Fig. 3. The entire skeleton, dorsal view with a scanning γ-camera 3 h after the injection of 19.0 mCi (703 MBq) of ^{99m}Tc-PP, in a male patient 50 years old, without neuplastic disease. See the more intense fixation in the axial skeleton and the homogeneous distribution in the vertebral column. (*B*, bladder activity.) The concentration is accentuated in the bones lying in the posterior plane because of the dorsal view

Fig. 4. Dorsal view of the skeleton by a large-head scanning γ-camera 4½ h after the injection of 20.2 mCi (748 MBq) ^{99m}Tc-MDP, in a 53-year-old woman with proven skeletal metastasis already present for 5 years, who was operated on for breast cancer 12 years before. Despite ovariectomy several courses of hormone- and chemotherapy, generalized skeletal relapse with metastatic involvement of all bones visualized. The differential diagnosis versus the homgeneous distribution encountered in a normal patient (see Fig. 3) is problematic. The scintigraphic aspect of the limbs, the heterogeneous distribution of MDP in the ribs, comparison with earlier scintigraphic findings, and quantitative analysis (standardized bone-to-soft tissue ratio) can help to establish the correct diagnosis

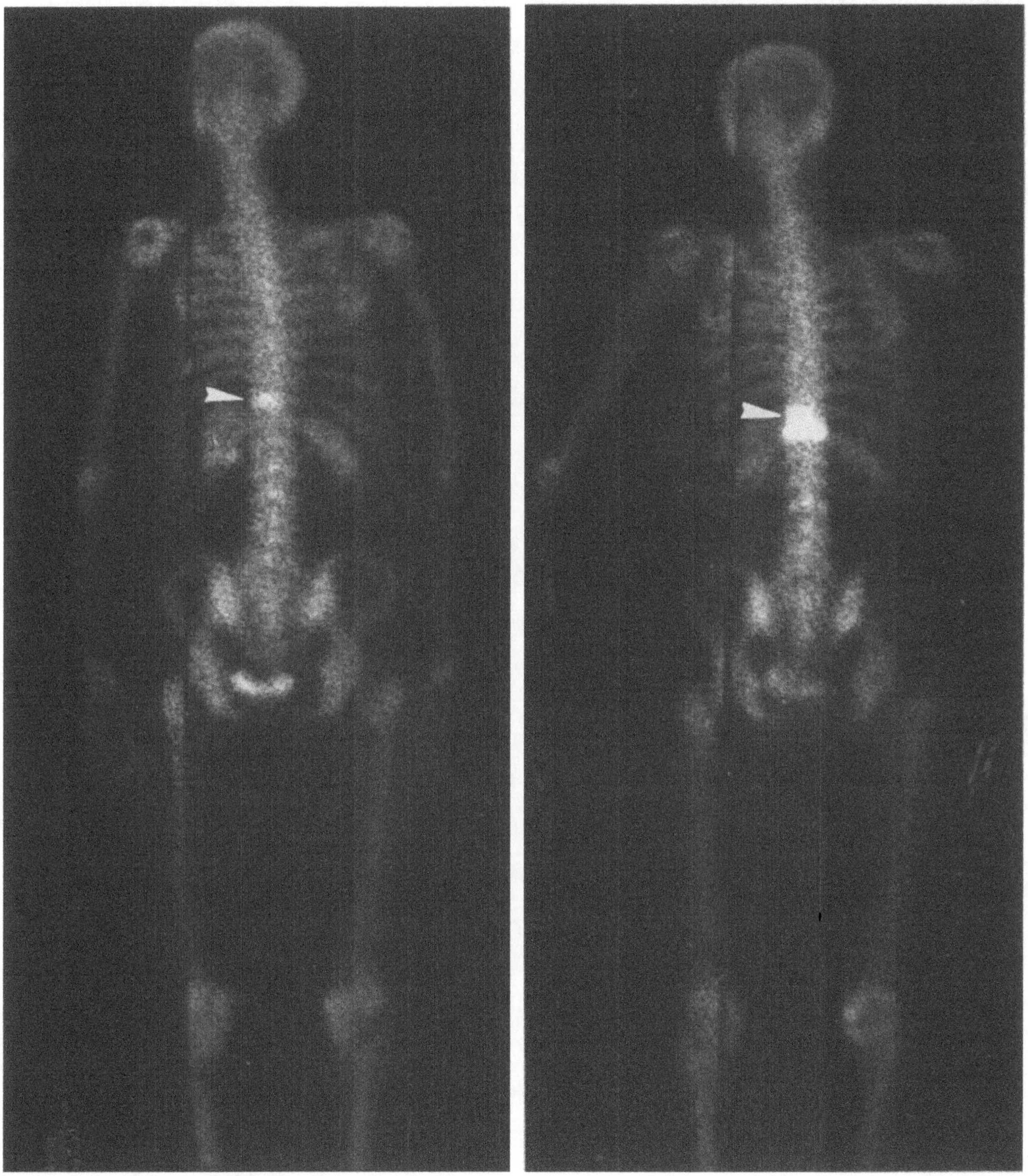

Fig. 5. a Isolated metastatic lesion involving T11 (*arrow*) in a 76-year-old woman with breast cancer (stage III) treated by surgery and x-ray therapy 6 years before. x-ray finding positive; **b** Scintigraphic control 1 year later: despite local radiotherapy pathologic image (*arrow*) involving T11 and T12. (For technical conditions of scintigraphy, see Fig. 4)

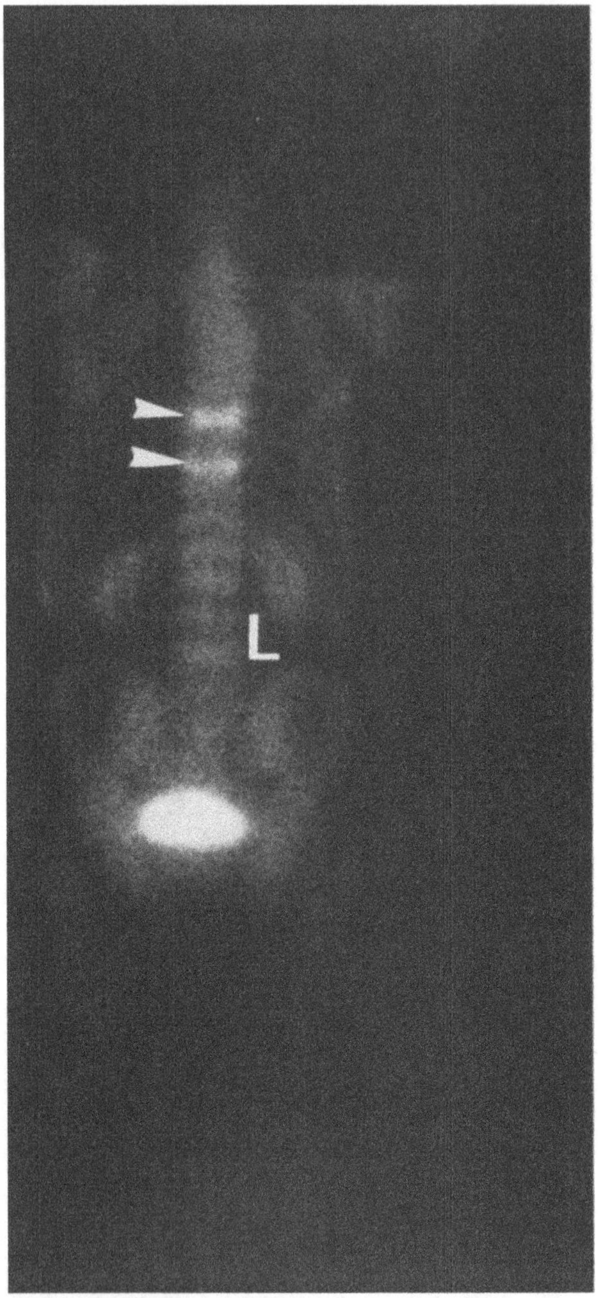

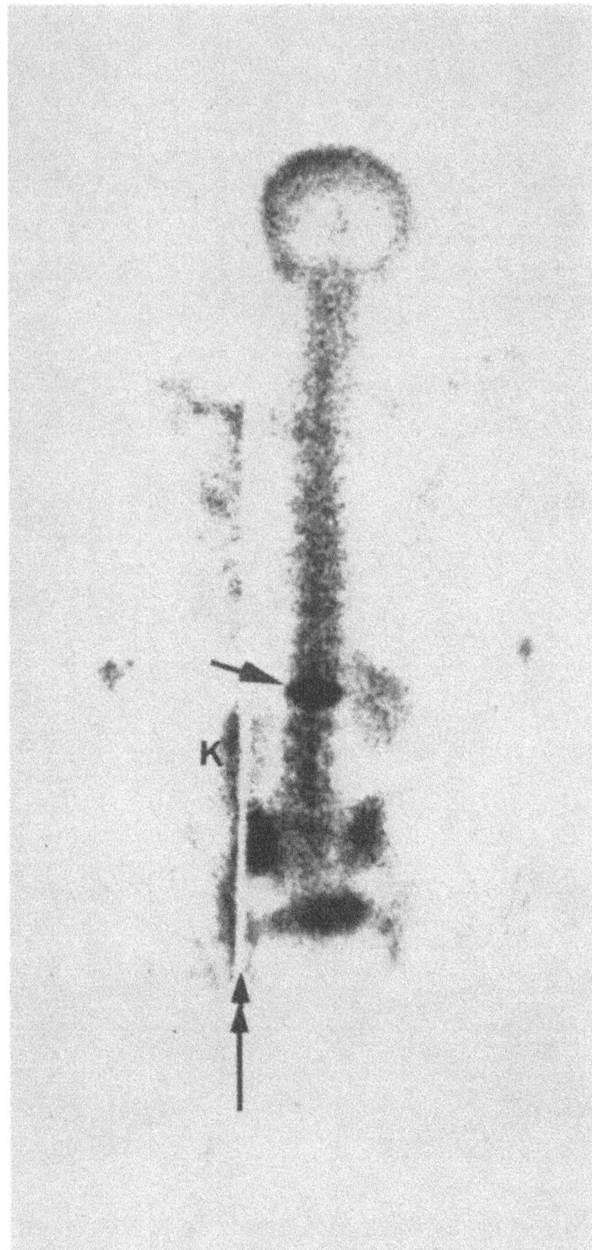

Fig. 6. Male patient, 71 years old, with carcinoma of the left lung treated by with several courses of chemotherapy for 16 months and back pain of recent onset in the thoracic section. Multiple pathologic involvement of the thoracic spine (*arrows*) and suggestive image of the lumbar spine (*L*). Standard x-ray examination 2 weeks later revealing metastatic involvement of several (lower thoracic and lumbar) vertebrae. Scintigram performed 5½ h after injection of 19.8 mCi (733 MBq) ^{99m}Tc-MDP in dorsal view with the same apparatus as used for examinations illustrated in the previous figures

Fig. 7. Cancer of the right tonsil (T4 No Mo) following 2 months' chemotherapy in a 55-year-old woman. Metastatic involvement of L2 (*arrow*) characterized by single localized focus of hyperfixation. Ptosis of the right kidney (*k*). Since the photographic contrast is accentuated, only the bones of the posterior part of the body are visualized. The *white line* (*double arrow*) corresponds to the electronic "soldering" of the pictures obtained from the two passes of the scanning γ-camera head. Scintigram performed 4 h after injection of the tracer (20 mCi ^{99m}Tc-MDP)

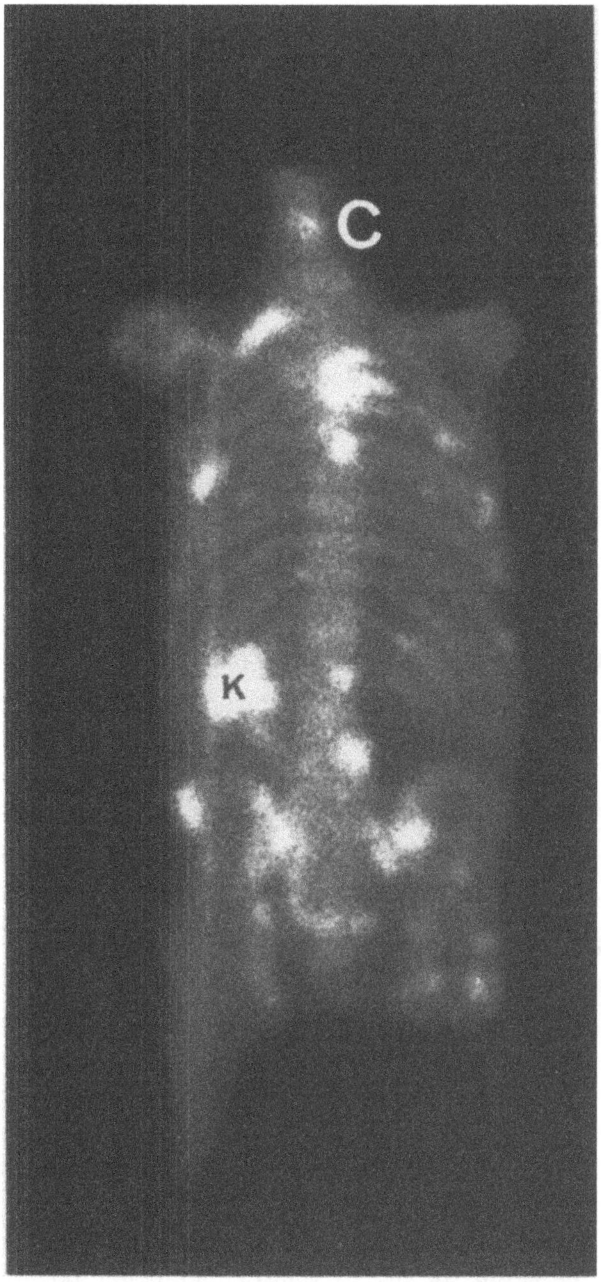

Fig. 8. Characteristic appearance of severe osseous involvement ("metastases in the spine and elsewhere") in a 79-year-old male patient with inoperable cancer of the rectum. There are several pathologic foci in all bones visualized, involving the cervical (*C*) thoracic and lumbar segments. Right hydronephrosis (*K*). Dorsal view of the skeleton recorded 2½ h after injection of 20.3 mCi (751 MBq) ^{99m}Tc-MDP

A great deal has already been written about RBI in the detection of bone metastases in various cancerous diseases [3, 5, 8, 14, 15, 22, 32], but a critical evaluation of all these papers is not the purpose of the present contribution. The reader is referred to the bibliographies in three recent works cited [3, 22, 32] for papers bearing on the detailed analysis of RBI in different neoplastic conditions. Our present purpose was to analyze, in identical technical conditions (labeled agents and apparatus used; person who established the findings), the metastatic involvement of the spine in the cancers most frequently encountered in daily clinical practice, and to study their distribution in the different segments of the vertebral column. The sacrum, which is embryologically and anatomically an integral part of the spine, has not been considered in this work, because (a) it is closely connected with the pelvis in its function; (b) none of the papers except two [2, 34], which deal with the same topic as the present chapter, deal with the sacrum (or the coccyx) and so, to preserve the possibility of comparative analysis with the data displayed in Table 2, we also limited our study to the three main segments of the vertebral column proper; and (c) since the spatial resolution in bone scintigraphy is sometimes problematic, it would often be rather difficult to determine precisely whether a pathologic focus belongs to the sacrum or to the pelvis. From the technical point of view it should also be borne in mind that pathologic lesions can occur in the vertebrae not only as hyperactive "hot spots" but also as hypoactive "cold zones" in the rare cases of a presumed metastatic embolus in the artery supplying a particular vertebra. This kind of lesion was identified in 2 cases among the 1036 patients with proven bone metastases in our population.

From the clinical point of view, as pointed out earlier, each case was recorded as metastatic or not according to the last verified scintiscan. For this reason, even when the differences in the percentage of verified global bone metastatic involvement are characteristic among the different cancers examined, the absolute values can be slightly lower when nonselected groups are studied. This is because our institute is a specialized cancer hospital and several patients had been treated in other institutions during the initial phase of their disease, only coming to our hospital when generalization was suspected. Precisely for this reason we did not analyze the metastatic involvement according to the clinical staging of a given cancer and did not establish the time lapse before the onset of bone metastases in the different categories. However, we did analyze relatively large and significant groups from the aspect of the proportion of spinal versus nonvertebral metastatic bone involvement and the intravertebral distribution of metastases in the case of both single and multiple pathologic localizations.

Even the figures in Table 1 demonstrate the high metastatic involvement encountered in the spine during the final evolution of several cancers. These results — which are taken from autopsy studies — were confirmed by those obtained in vivo by scintigraphic examination either by other authors (see Table 2) or by ourselves. These data underline, if still necessary, the importance of the vertebral venous circulation, which constitutes a preferential route for metastatic cells, as demonstrated experimentally by BATSON [4] to explain the high percentage of spinal bone metastases encountered in most cancerous diseases studied. Perhaps the most original statement possible on the basis of the analysis of our patients is that there is a cervical-to-lumbar gradient for spinal metastatic involvement, expressed as an increasing percentage of metastases per vertebra, and that this is true for all the patients studied, whether they had single or multiple spinal metastases. This can be explained only by the lumbar-to-cervical venous current in the valveless network, providing the preferential route of spread, especially in the case of increased intra-abdominal pressure [4, 14]. The greater size of lumbar vertebrae and the higher local venous blood flow may also contribute to the higher incidence of metastatic involvement in lumbar vertebrae.

Analysis of the data displayed in Fig. 1 allows some interesting statements about the differences in spinal localization of bone metastases among the selected neoplastic diseases studied. It is not surprising that prostatic and breast carcinoma are accompanied by the highest incidence of bone involvement in general; it is more interesting that all six other cancers present approximately the same incidence of metastatic bone involvement regardless of their relatively different histological nature, at least in the given conditions of similar patient selection. As pointed out previously, the breast and prostatic cancers do not only have the highest degree of metastatic bone involvement, but also the most significant participation of the spine in the bone involvement, with less than 20% metastases at other sites than in the vertebrae. Invasion of the whole body by circulating cancerous cells originating from the prostate could take place directly by way of the vertebral venous system, as demonstrated by BATSON experimentally [4]. Since the breast is connected directly to the same venous system by the segmental veins of the chest wall [4, 14], the high incidence of vertebral involvement also seems logical in mammary carcinoma. The same mechanism could also explain the significant incidence of spinal involvement (75% of all bone metastases), encountered in lung cancer patients.

On the other hand, three neoplastic diseases, lymphomas, melanomas, and cancers of the head and neck exhibit a specific behavior characterized by a relatively lower involvement (53%–54%) of the spine by metastatic bone disease. The specific nature of lymphomas as a systemic disease, the generalized localization of melanomas, and the mandatory loco-regional lymphatic passage of the squamous cell carcinomas of the head and neck region might explain how during the initial invasive phase of metastatic disease a large proportion of neoplastic cells might escapes to the vertebral venous circulation. Moreover, in this group, when the spine is affected by metastatic bone disease single vertebral foci are most usual, a further indication of lower susceptibility to vertebral localization.

From the point of view of the natural history of the neoplastic disease and of therapeutic policy, vertebral metastases might have an important role insofar as they might predispose to future fractures, with all their direct complications, or give rise to creeping infiltration toward the vertebral canal, the meninges, or the spinal cord, with extremely severe clinical and neurologic consequences. For this reason it is important to know for sure whether there is metastatic bone disease of the spine and if so, its precise localization. These data seem to represent specific characteristics of all neoplastic diseases studied, at least according to the results discussed in this chapter, and should be taken into account during the initial staging and in selection of the treatment policy.

As a clinically useful method, RBI plays a decisive role in the search of vertebral bone metastases, the high sensitivity of the method unfortunately being partly offset by a tendencey to give false-positive images. This technique of nuclear medicine can doubtless be improved on in the future by more extensive application of computer-assisted quantitative evaluation of scintigrams [1, 10, 11, 27], by the wider availability of SPECT-type cameras, by the introduction of newer bone-seeking agents with higher bone/soft tissue and metastase/normal bone ratios, and perhaps by application of the radioimmunoscintigraphic technique [21]. On the other hand, the combined use of the main medical imaging techniques (scintigraphy, conventional radiology, CT scan) is particularly recommended [5, 18] and should reduce the percentages of false positives and negatives, whereas the future role of NMR imaging still needs to be precisely specified in the field of bone pathology.

E. Summary and Conclusions

The incidence, the anatomic localization, and the segmental distribution in the spine of positive scintigraphic bone lesions have been studied in 1036 patients with proven metastatic bone involvement deriving from histologically demonstrated neoplastic disease. The analysis of the data obtained led to the following statements:

Prostatic and breast cancers are accompanied by the highest percentage of metastatic bone disease and also the most significant involvement of the spine (80%–89% of all metastases identified).

Three kinds of neoplastic disease (lymphomas, melanomas, head and neck cancers) involve a relatively substantial proportion of bone metastases (46%–47%) localized elsewhere than in the vertebral column.

In most cases when vertebral bone metastases are present these are combined with pathologic localizations elsewhere; the incidence of isolated spinal involvement remains under 10% in all groups except lung carcinoma.

Consideration of single and multiple vertebral metastases separately shows that the general incidence of the first group is only 12%. In any given cancer, the lower the incidence of spinal metastasis in general, the higher the number of cases with only one vertebral focus.

Of all metastatic foci, 16.1% were identified in the cervical segment, 45.9% in thoracic vertebrae, and 38 in the lumbar spine, revealing a "top-to-bottom gradient," the incidences as percentages of metastatic foci/single vertebra being 2.29 for the cervical, 3.82 for the thoracic, and 7.61 for the lumbar region.

The high incidence of spinal metastatic disease, the differences encountered in the various groups examined, and the existence of the above-mentioned gradient underline the important role of the vertebral venous system in the etiology and distribution of metastatic bone involvement.

References

1. Anger K (1980) Die quantitative Ganzkörper-Skelettszintigraphie. Nuklearmedizin 19:64–73; 97–107; 108–109
2. Aufses AH (1930) Skeletal metastases from carcinoma of the rectum; report of 8 cases. Arch Surg 21:916–923
3. Basset LW, Gold RH, Webber MM (1981) Radionuclide bone imaging. Radiol Clin North Am 19:675–702
4. Batson OV (1981) The vertebral vein system (Caldwell Lecture, 1956). In: Weiss L, Gilbert HA (eds) Bone metastasis. Hall, Boston, pp 21–48
5. De Wilde A, Frühling J, Osteaux M, Jeanmart L, Henry J (1976) Confrontation des résultats de la scintigraphie osseouse et de la radiographie systématique du squelette dans la recherche des métastases au cours de l'évolution des néoplasies mammaires. J Belge Radiol 59:131–138
6. Drury AB, Palmer PH, Higham WJ (1964) Carcinomatous metastasis to the vertebral bodies. J Clin Pathol 17:448–457
7. Eggenstein G, Drochmans A, De Roo M, Wildiers J, Devos P, Van Der Schueren G (1978) Bone scintigraphy as detection method for bone and bone marrow involvement in malignant lymphoma with regard to other exploration techniques. J Belge Radiol 61:471–480
8. Ell PJ, Dash J, Raymond J (1976) Bone scanning; a review on purpose and method. Skeletal Radiol 1:33–45
9. Fihn SD, Larson EB, Rudd TR, Nelp WB (1982) Clinical use of radionuclide bone imaging in a University Medical Center. JAMA 248:439–442
10. Fogelman J, Bessent R, Scullion JE, Cuthbert, GF (1982) Accuracy of 24-h whole body (skeletal) retention of diphosphate measurements. Eur J Nucl Med 7:359–363
11. Fogelman J, Martin W (1983) Assessment of skeletal uptake of ^{99m}Tc-Diphosphonate over a five day period. Eur J Nucl Med 8:489–490
12. Fon GT, Wong WS, Gold RM, Kaiser LR (1981) Skeletal metastases of melanoma: radiographic, scintigraphic and clinical review. AJR 137:103–108

13. Galasko CSB (1972) Skeletal metastases and mammary cancer. Ann R Coll Surg Engl 50:3–28
14. Galasko CSB (1981) The anatomy and pathways of skeletal metastases. In: Weiss L, Gilbert HA (eds) Bone metastasis. Hall, Boston, pp 49–63
15. Galasko CSB (1981) The development of skeletal metastases. In: Weiss L, Gilbert HA (eds) Bone metastasis. Hall, Boston, pp 83–113
16. Holmes FF, Fouts TL (1970) Metastatic cancer of unknown primary site. Cancer 26:816–820
17. Kaufmann E (1902) Pathologische Anatomie der malignen Neoplasmen der Prostata. Dtsch. J Chir 53:381
18. Lenz M, Freid JR (1931) Metastases to skeleton, brain and spinal cord from cancer of the breast and effect of radiotherapy. Ann Surg 93:278–293
19. Levenson RM, Sauerbrunn BJL, Bates HR, Newmann RD, Eddy JL, Ihde DC (1983) Comparative value of bone scintigraphy and radiography in monitoring tumor response in systematically treated prostatic carcinoma. Radiology 146:513–518
20. Liedholm A, Lundell L, Martenson B, Thulin A (1978) Skeletal scintigraphy in the initial assessment of woman with breast cancer. Acta Chir Scand 145:65–71
21. Mach JP, Carrel S, Forni M, Ritschard J, Donath A, Alberto P (1980) Tumor localization of radiolabeled antibodies against carcinoembryonic antigen in patients with carcinoma; a critical evaluation. N Engl J Med 303:5–10
22. Mahlstedt J, Schümichen C, Biersack HJ (1981) Skelettszintigraphie. Giebeler, Darmstadt, pp 1–87
23. Newcomer LN, Silverstein MB, Cadman EC, Farber LR, Bertino JR, Prosnitz LR (1982) Bone involvement in Hodgkin's disease. Cancer 49:338-342
24. Nomura Y, Kondo H, Yamagata Y, Kanda K, Takenaka K, Maeda T, Shiokawa H (1978) Evaluation of liver and bone scanning in patients with early breast cancer, based on results obtained from more advanced cancer patients. Eur J Cancer 14:1129–1136
25. Pagani JJ, Libschitz HJ (1982) Imaging bone metastases. Radiol Clin North Am 20:545–560
26. Pauwels EKJ, Blom J, Camps JAJ, Hermans J, Rijke AM (1983) A comparison between the diagnostic efficacy of ^{99m}Tc-DPD and ^{99m}Tc-HDP for the detection of bone metastases. Eur J Nucl Med 8:118–122
27. Pecking A, Delorme G, Deband B, Gest J (1983) Métastases osseuse du cancer du sein. Intérêt diagnostique et prévisionnel de la scintigraphie osseouse quantifiée. Presse Med 12:1215–1218
28. Pürckhauer R (1929) Das Prostatacarcinom; seine Häufigkeit und seine Metastasen. Z Krebsforsch 28:68–95
29. Rampon S, Bussiere J-J, Prin Ph, Sauvezie B, Leroy V, Missioux D, Doly J, Suss P, Jourde H, Lapalus P (1974) A propos de 250 observations de scintigraphie osseuse par le pyrophosphate d'étain marqué au technétium 99m. Revue du Rhumatisme (Paris) 41:745–751
30. Simpson WM (1926) Primary thyroid carcinoma simulating hypernephroma. Am Clin Med 4:668–672
31. Wahner HW, Kyle RA, Beabout JW (1980) Scintigraphic evaluation of the skeleton in multiple myeloma. Mayo Clin Proc 55:739–746
32. Weiss L, Gilbert HA (eds) (1981) Bone metastasis. Hall, Boston
33. Wiebe V, Erbe W (1973) Skelettmetastasen differenzierter Schilddrüsenkarzinome – Röntgenbild, Szintigramm, Verlauf unter Behandlund. RoFo 118:313–319
34. Willis RA (1973) The spread of tumours in the human body, 3rd ed Butterworths, London
35. Wilson MA, Calhoun FW (1981) The distribution of skeletal metastases in breast and pulmunary cancer: concise communication. J Nucl Med 22:594–597

Subject Index

www.ingramcontent.com/pod-product-compliance
Lightning Source LLC
Chambersburg PA
CBHW061220240926
51846CB00006B/1294
* 9 7 8 3 6 4 2 4 9 3 0 5 8 *